THE ANTI-ANXIETY WORKBOOK

THE GUILFORD SELF-HELP WORKBOOK SERIES
Martin M. Antony, Series Editor

Workbooks in this series are crafted by respected scientists who are also seasoned therapists. Each volume addresses a specific psychological or emotional problem, putting powerful change strategies directly into the reader's hands. Special features include self-assessment tools, worksheets, skills-building exercises, and examples—plus the support and motivation readers need to achieve their goals.

**The Anti-Anxiety Workbook: Proven Strategies
to Overcome Worry, Phobias, Panic, and Obsessions**
Martin M. Antony and Peter J. Norton

The
Anti-Anxiety
Workbook

Proven Strategies to Overcome
Worry, Phobias, Panic, and Obsessions

Martin M. Antony
Peter J. Norton

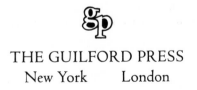

THE GUILFORD PRESS
New York   London

© 2009 The Guilford Press
A Division of Guilford Publications, Inc.
72 Spring Street, New York, NY 10012
www.guilford.com

Printed in the United States of America

This book is printed on acid-free paper.

Last digit is print number: 9 8 7 6 5 4 3 2 1

Library of Congress Cataloging-in-Publication Data

Antony, Martin M.
    The anti-anxiety workbook : proven strategies to overcome worry, phobias, panic, and obsessions / Martin M. Antony, Peter J. Norton.
        p.   cm. — (The Guilford self-help workbook series)
    Includes bibliographical references and index.
    ISBN 978-1-59385-993-0 (pbk. : alk. paper)
    1. Anxiety disorders—Treatment—Popular works.   I. Norton, Peter J.,
1972–   II. Title.
    RC531.A554 2009
    616.85′22—dc22
                                                            2008026718

*While writing this book, I also had the pleasure of helping to launch
new master's and PhD programs in psychology at Ryerson University
in Toronto. I dedicate this book to our first class of graduate students.*
—M. M. A.

For my family
—P. J. N.

Acknowledgments

We would like to thank our editors at The Guilford Press, Kitty Moore and Linda Carbone, for their guidance and encouragement throughout the process. Thanks also to Drs. Lakshmi Ravindran, Richard Swinson, and Mark Watling for their thoughtful comments and suggestions regarding the chapter on medication treatments. A special thank you to those who first developed, shaped, and studied many of the strategies described in this book, as well as to our mentors, who first exposed us to these approaches: David H. Barlow, Aaron T. Beck, Thomas Borkovec, Timothy A. Brown, David M. Clark, Michelle G. Craske, Hans Eysenck, Edna B. Foa, Steven Hayes, Richard G. Heimberg, Debra Hope, Isaac Marks, Ron Norton, Lars-Goran Öst, Randy Paterson, S. Rachman, Ron Rapee, Paul Salkovskis, Richard Swinson, Maureen Whittal, Joseph Wolpe, and many others.

Contents

Introduction: The Faces of Anxiety   I

PART I

The Prep

1. *Anxiety: The Big Picture*   7

2. *Getting to Know Your Anxiety*   35

3. *Getting Ready for Treatment*   58

PART II

The Program

4. *Changing Your Anxious Thinking*   79

5. *Eliminating the Safety Net*   107

6. *Confronting Feared Objects and Situations*   125

7. *Confronting Scary Thoughts, Memories, Images, and Urges*   136

8. *Confronting Frightening Feelings and Sensations*   148

9. *Learning to Relax: Relaxation, Meditation, and Acceptance*   157

10. *Medications and Herbal Remedies*   171

PART III

In the Long Run

11. *Creating an Anti-Anxiety Lifestyle*　　　　　　　195

12. *Overcoming Treatment Obstacles*　　　　　　　207

13. *Living without Anxiety*　　　　　　　　　　221

14. *A Guide for Family and Friends*　　　　　　234

Appendix: Helpful Resources　　　　　　　　243

Index　　　　　　　　　　　　　　　257

About the Authors　　　　　　　　　　262

Introduction
The Faces of Anxiety

Valerie paces around her apartment as she waits for her husband to arrive home from work. It's 6:00 P.M., and she wonders where he is. She tried calling him on his cell phone, but there was no answer. He normally finishes work at 5:00 P.M., and it only takes him about a half hour to get home. Her mind starts to race. What's making him late? Perhaps he's been in a terrible accident, she thinks. Maybe he's gotten fired and is drinking himself into a stupor at some bar. Could it be an affair? Valerie feels her emotions swing from worry to anger to terror. She's frustrated because there's nothing she can do but wait. About a half hour later, Carl walks in the door, explaining that there'd been construction on the highway and the traffic was backed up. Why hadn't he answered his cell phone? Simple: he didn't have it with him. Indeed, Valerie now notices it lying on an end table. She breathes a sigh of relief. As she often does, Valerie had let her anxiety get the best of her.

Don is terrified of flying. Most of the time he avoids planes completely. Once in a while, though, he will take a short flight if he absolutely has to. When he does, he purposely stays awake the night before so he'll be more likely to sleep on the plane. He also has a few drinks on the flight, and may even take a Valium (which he doesn't know is a potentially dangerous combination). He does everything he can to distract himself when he's not sleeping, including reading, listening to music, and talking to the person sitting next to him. If he has to fly, he starts worrying about it months in advance. Nightmares often invade his dreams. Because of his fear of a plane crash, he has turned down promotions, avoided vacations, and even missed his parents' 40th wedding anniversary celebration.

Jacqui is a new mom. Although she has never had significant problems with anxiety in the past, she now finds she has intrusive thoughts about harming her newborn daughter. For example, when changing her baby's diaper, she sometimes experiences thoughts of strangling or sexually abusing her daughter. The thoughts shock and scare her. She has no desire to do these things and would never act on the thoughts, but she worries that they're a sign that she might do something bad to her daughter or that she's a terrible mother. Jacqui knows such thoughts aren't normal, and she does everything she can to avoid thinking them. She tries not to be alone with her baby or to be around anything that could be used to hurt her baby (for example, knives). But the more she tries not to think about hurting her baby, the more upset she becomes when experiencing intrusive thoughts.

Jacob worries about his health. When he was a teenager, his father suddenly collapsed from a stroke and died in the hospital. While Jacob was at the hospital with his father, he saw many other stroke patients, some of whom couldn't speak, were partially paralyzed, or seemed like "vegetables." Ever since then, Jacob has been terrified of having a stroke or some other sudden major health problem. Whenever Jacob experiences a sharp headache, he immediately fears that he's having a stroke or an aneurysm. Terrified that he will die, Jacob rushes to the emergency room. Each time, the doctors run some tests and assure him that he isn't dying, and then he feels lucky, as though he has cheated death. But each time he also worries that the next time might really be a stroke.

What do Valerie, Don, Jacqui, and Jacob have in common? Each of them experiences excessive or exaggerated anxiety and fear. Valerie never even considers many common possibilities for her husband's delay. Don's fear of flying persists even though flying is actually one of the safest ways to travel (the most dangerous part of a flight is the drive to the airport!). Jacqui is terrified of her own thoughts, even though she knows she would never act on them. Jacob is convinced that his physical sensations are signs of an impending stroke, even though he is in excellent health.

These are the faces of anxiety. Sometimes it's easy to understand how anxiety begins, as with Jacob, whose anxiety developed while he watched his father die from a stroke. Other times, the anxiety may seem absurd or difficult to understand, like Jacqui's thoughts about harming her infant. Everyone experiences anxiety and fear from time to time, but for some of us, the anxiety and fear take control. These emotions dictate what we can and can't do. These emotions fire us up, even when everyone else around us would say there's no cause for concern.

This book is written for people who experience anxiety and fear in this way. Here you'll learn the most widely studied and accepted techniques that mental health professionals use for helping people overcome problems of extreme anxiety. The chapters are organized to simulate the steps that an experienced therapist would take you through. Part I is "The Prep." First, we'll teach you what anxiety is and why yours has grown out of control. Then we'll guide you through a self-assessment to openly and honestly take stock of how anxiety affects you and your life. Although this workbook is for a wide audience of anxiety sufferers, it's carefully designed to help readers develop a treatment plan designed specifically for them. In Chapter 3, we will show you how to use the results of your self-assessments to plan your own treatment, tailoring the techniques presented in this book to your particular fears and worries.

Chapters 4 through 10 ("The Program") present the core of the treatment, which is based on an approach known as cognitive-behavioral therapy, or CBT. CBT is, by far, the most widely accepted, studied, and proven psychological treatment for helping people overcome their fears. You will start by learning to identify the thoughts and assumptions that are driving your fears and to practice techniques that will allow you to shift your anxious thoughts to a more realistic place. With these skills, you can begin to confront the situations that trigger your fear and anxiety. Don't be afraid! This will be a gradual process conducted at a manageable pace. Just work through the beginning sections of the book and practice the skills we recommend, and you'll be ready to confront the situations that give rise to your anxieties. In addition, you'll learn techniques to help you relax and control the physical manifestations of your anxiety. In Chapter 10, you'll also learn how medications can be used to reduce your anxiety symptoms.

In the last few chapters of this book, "In the Long Run," we offer ways to help cement the changes you've made while working through this program: strategies for preventing your anxiety from returning, techniques for overcoming barriers that occasionally get in the way of recovery, and personal changes you can make for an anxiety-free lifestyle. We wrote the last chapter specifically for your loved ones. As we have seen over and over again, our partners, family members, and friends can be our biggest source of support or (sometimes) our biggest barrier to recovery. This chapter provides your family and friends with a better appreciation of what you've been going through and gives them their own skills for helping you on your journey toward overcoming anxiety.

Recommendations for Working Through This Program

Feel free to use this book in whatever way you think will be most helpful to you, but we do have some tips for how to get the most out of this treatment program. We recommend that you first skim through the entire book before applying the techniques and skills we describe. We want you to be familiar not only with the ideas and skills each chapter presents but also with the treatment program as a whole. This program is designed to build upon the techniques you have learned and advances you have made in earlier sections, so it's important for you to see the "big picture" as you practice using particular strategies.

In addition, we would like you to flag Chapter 12 so that you can refer to it easily. This is the one chapter that's meant to be consulted out of order as you practice the strategies from the earlier parts of the book. Chapter 12 is about dealing with problems that sometimes arise while you're working through the program. This is where you should turn when you feel that something isn't working. It will give you ideas and suggestions when you can't seem to fit your recovery into your hectic schedule. The types of treatment obstacles that are discussed in Chapter 12 include:

+ Difficulty finding the time for treatment (for example, to complete homework practices)
+ Coping with other psychological problems, such as depression or substance abuse
+ Difficulty getting motivated
+ Life stress (at work, in relationships, or in other areas)
+ Medical complications
+ Lack of relevant skills (for example, communication skills, driving skills)

We hope that you will make the necessary commitment to immerse yourself fully in the steps outlined in this book for letting go of your anxiety, fear, phobias, obsessions, and compulsions. These techniques work! That's been proven time and time again by scientists in controlled studies, by therapists in their work with patients, and by people just like you. But it doesn't happen by looking at words on a page. It will only happen by taking the ideas and recommendations on these pages and putting them into action in your life.

Through no fault of your own, anxiety has been telling you what you can and can't do. It has closed doors and restricted the pleasure you experience every day. It has taken away important parts of your life. *Turn the page and begin to take back your life.*

PART I

The Prep

1

Anxiety
The Big Picture

You're one of the millions of people who have an anxiety disorder, but with the right help you can overcome it. You've taken an important step by beginning this book. Maybe you already know a lot about the different kinds of anxiety disorders and even know the name of exactly which one you suffer from. Or maybe all these terms will be new to you. Either way, before you start *The Anti-Anxiety Workbook* program, it's a good idea to build a general understanding of just what anxiety is and how it can be tamed.

Just as someone with heart disease or high blood pressure needs to comprehend the nature of the illness and get the right medical help, you need to get on the right track to rid yourself of the burden you've been carrying that has kept you from being the person you want to be—at work, at home, and in social situations. This chapter gives you a good grasp of the fundamentals: the nature of anxiety, the main types of anxiety disorders, the triggers for anxiety, its causes, and its effective treatments. In the next chapter, we take a more tailored view of your particular anxiety once you have a broad base to put it in some context.

Let's start with the concept that anxiety is a universal emotion experienced by everyone everywhere—probably even by most animals. We need our anxiety. It does us a lot of good in many situations. But when it's out of our control—as you know all too well—it does us harm. In fact, as hard as it may be to believe, the anxiety and fear systems in your body are probably working in exactly the way they were designed to work. They are just going off at the wrong times, just like when the smoke detector in your home sometimes goes off when you are cooking. The smoke detector is doing what it is designed to do—but at the wrong time. But what exactly are fear and anxiety?

What Is Anxiety?

Anxiety occurs when you're confronted with a possible threat, danger, or negative event, particularly something over which you have little control. When you feel anxious, your body becomes aroused. You may experience muscle tension, increased heart rate, and other physical changes. Your attention also becomes more focused—on the possible source of the threat as well as on your own functioning (for example, on your feelings of arousal). This process is designed to help you prevent or avoid possible danger in the future.

This focus of attention on the potential source of danger is called *hypervigilance*. Hypervigilance makes it hard for you to concentrate on your work or on other normal activities such as reading or having a conversation. You may also start to *worry*, which involves trying to think about possible plans or solutions to disarm the perceived threat. Finally, anxiety is often associated with *avoidance*. When you're anxious, you may try to avoid situations that you perceive as threatening. You may also try to avoid your own experiences—in particular, the physical sensations and anxiety-provoking thoughts that accompany your negative emotions.

Parker is a good example of what happens to us when we feel anxious. A 19-year-old college student, she has an exam tomorrow in her second-year calculus class. She hasn't studied at all. She needs to do well on this exam because she did poorly on the last one. Parker's anxiety level is very high when she thinks about the exam—so high, in fact, that she can't concentrate on studying. She can't help but focus on how uncomfortable she feels and how bad it will be if she doesn't get a good grade.

She tries to think of ways to concentrate better, but she simply can't. Finally, she gives up and decides to go to sleep. She figures that at least she'll be well rested if not well prepared for the test. Unfortunately, the more she tries to fall asleep, the more aroused and awake she feels. No attempt to distract herself from her anxiety works. Her worry keeps her awake the whole night.

Clearly, Parker is experiencing anxiety—a negative emotion focused on the possibility of future threat (in this case, an exam). The good news is that the strategies described in this book have helped countless individuals just like Parker to overcome their anxiety and get on with their lives.

Anxiety versus Fear

Unlike anxiety, which is focused on some *future* threat, fear is an intense emotional reaction to some *immediate* threat or danger. Helen fears snakes, for example, and experiences anxiety about possibly encountering one whenever she goes to the pet store to pick up food for her hamster. One day she actually saw a snake at the pet store, which triggered fear—her entire behavior was focused on getting out of the store as quickly as possible. Anxiety zeroes in on possible future dangers, while fear is focused on the here and now. It deals with immediate and real dangers, as well as with perceived dangers that only seem immediate and real.

Fear activates your somatic nervous system in order to prepare you to face danger.

Your body's response to immediate danger is often referred to as the "fight-or-flight response" because all the changes in your body are designed to help you respond to the threat with either an aggressive response (fight) or an escape from the situation (flight).

You may not think of it this way, but anger is also a response to potential threat. Think about the last time you felt very angry about something. What triggered it? What did you feel like just before you got angry? Chances are that just before feeling angry, you felt hurt, vulnerable, or threatened in some way. Understanding that anxiety and anger are both responses to potential threat helps explain why people with anxiety disorders often display high levels of anger and irritability.

This book focuses mostly on the "flight" side of the fight-or-flight response (in other words, fear), as opposed to the "fight" side (anger). Fear is the sort of response you might experience if a growling dog was chasing you, if you were being mugged at gunpoint, or if you were traveling in a car with a reckless driver, narrowly dodging one serious accident after another. When you're afraid, your body becomes mobilized for action. Your heart may start to race or pound. Your breathing rate increases. You may also experience sweating, dizziness, and many other symptoms of arousal. Fear is also associated with a strong urge to perform some action to reduce the potential threat. Most often, that action involves escape, avoidance, or engaging in some sort of safety behavior to ward it off.

The Relationship between Fear and Anxiety

We all feel fear and anxiety from time to time. But if you have an anxiety disorder, you feel these emotions frequently. You may find that you have difficulty labeling your own emotions, or that terms such as "anxiety" and "fear" don't seem to capture what you feel. What terms do you use to describe the feelings that led you to start reading this book? Perhaps more general terms such as "discomfort" or "uneasiness" seem closer to what you experience. States such as terror or panic are probably more closely related to fear. Apprehension, nervousness, and worry are probably more closely related to anxiety. Pick the descriptions that seem right to you. Regardless of what words you use to describe these states, the strategies in this book can help you overcome them.

The Benefits of Anxiety and Fear

You may be surprised to learn that anxiety and fear serve a useful function. Surely you find anxiety and fear unpleasant, but you wouldn't want to be entirely rid of them. You *need* them in order to survive. As you just learned, anxiety is designed to help you prepare for a *possible* future threat; fear is designed to help you escape in the face of some *immediate* threat. Just as you might adjust the sensitivity of the smoke detector so that it stops blaring when you are cooking, your goal here is to adjust your anxiety and fear so that they turn on only when they're appropriate to the situation.

The relationship between anxiety and performance is complex. People often assume that anxiety leads to impaired performance at work, at school, and in other activities, but it's not that simple. In fact, at low levels, anxiety has exactly the opposite effect, actually seeming to improve functioning and performance. Think about it. Many of the things you do on a day-to-day basis are inspired by your concern about the possible consequences of *not* doing these things; in other words, they're motivated by anxiety. You drive within the speed limit to avoid getting a ticket or being in an accident; you arrive at work on time each day to avoid being fired; you pay your bills to avoid the potential legal and financial consequences of not paying them.

Low to moderate levels of anxiety actually provide you with the motivation to get things done. If you had no anxiety, chances are that many necessary tasks would never be completed. You might even be inclined to do things that are impulsive and risky. For example, there is evidence that people who engage in criminal behavior may respond to particular threatening situations with less anxiety and fear than people who are not inclined toward antisocial behavior. It may be that anxiety about getting caught contributes to preventing some people from committing crimes.

Although low to moderate levels of anxiety motivate us to work hard and perform well, high levels can interfere with our ability to get things done. If you're making a big presentation at work, a moderate level of anxiety might keep you on your toes. But extreme anxiety would make it difficult for you to concentrate, thereby increasing the chances that you would lose your train of thought and botch parts of your presentation. The goal of this book, then, is not to rid you of all anxiety but to help you achieve levels of anxiety that enhance your performance, rather than getting in its way.

Like anxiety, fear also has important benefits. Fear is designed to protect you from immediate danger. When you feel fear, your body goes into overdrive. Your heart rate increases to push more blood to your large muscles to facilitate escape; your breathing rate increases to provide the extra oxygen your body needs to flee the situation; you sweat heavily to cool off your body so you can perform more efficiently. In fact, most of your body's responses during fear or panic make it easier for you to escape. Not only are the symptoms of fear and panic not dangerous (contrary to what many people believe when they are experiencing panic), but they are doing vital work to protect you from danger. Fear and panic are only a problem when they occur too frequently, too intensely, and in the absence of true danger, thereby preventing you from doing things that you want to do.

What Triggers Anxiety and Fear?

Anxiety and fear are reactions to perceived threat. This means essentially that we *interpret* a situation to be dangerous in some way. It doesn't mean that the situation *is* dangerous. Scary movies are a good example of this. We often feel afraid during the movie because it seems so realistic, but we aren't in any real danger of Hannibal Lecter coming out of the television and attacking us. Or you might be temporarily startled to come home and find the front door unlocked, then realize that your spouse came home early that day.

Anxiety and fear are almost always triggered by something. There are two main types of triggers: external and internal.

External Triggers

External triggers are objects, situations, or activities that we experience as threatening. For example, people with phobias may experience triggers in the form of heights, spiders, snakes, driving, flying, public speaking, or other things or situations. People who worry too much may become anxious when a loved one is late arriving home. People with concerns about germs may respond to triggers such as touching elevator buttons, doorknobs, or other objects in public places. People who fear slipping on the ice may avoid going out at all on very cold days.

In all these examples, the anxiety trigger is something external to the individual. It's a place or situation (for example, a high mountain), an activity (such as sitting on a public toilet), or an object (like a dog). If you believe an external trigger poses a threat, you're likely to deal with it by *avoidance* (turning down an invitation to a party because of anxiety in social situations), *escape* (leaving a party early due to anxiety), or *safety behaviors* (wearing extra makeup and a turtleneck sweater to a party to hide blushing on the face and neck).

Internal Triggers

Internal triggers for anxiety and fear are private, internal experiences that we experience as threatening. One type of internal trigger involves physical sensations and feelings (sometimes called *interoceptive* cues or triggers). Here are some examples in which these triggers play an important role:

- ✦ A woman with panic attacks is terrified that her racing heart could cause a heart attack. She panics whenever she notices the slightest increase in her heart rate even if she knows it's caused by something else, like exercise.
- ✦ A man with a fear of heights is terrified of feeling dizzy in high places, convinced that he will lose his balance and fall.
- ✦ A person with claustrophobia fears suffocating in enclosed places. The sensation of breathlessness triggers a panicky feeling, particularly when she feels closed in.
- ✦ Someone who is nervous in social situations is particularly frightened of having shaky hands. He's convinced that other people will notice his shakiness and view him as weak or incompetent.

Another type of internal trigger involves thoughts or imagery, often referred to as *cognitive* triggers (the word *cognitive* refers to mental processes such as thinking, memory, and attention). Just as people can be afraid of their physical sensations, they can fear their own mental experiences (such as thoughts, images, or urges). Consider these examples:

- ✦ A woman who was raped 5 years ago is still terrified when she thinks about that horrible event. She does everything she can to block the memories from entering her mind. She believes that if she allows herself to think about the rape, she may become so anxious that she will "go crazy" or lose control.

✦ A person with obsessive–compulsive disorder is terrified of having thoughts about hurting his loved ones, especially when such thoughts pop into his head unexpectedly. He knows he won't act on these thoughts, yet he feels compelled to keep them from entering his mind.

✦ A man who is fearful of vomiting does everything he can to avoid thinking of vomiting. Even the thought of vomiting arouses some nausea, and he fears that thinking about vomiting could cause it to happen.

People who react with fear and anxiety in response to internal triggers are often afraid of their emotions, particularly of feeling anxious or frightened, which is associated with the very sensations, thoughts, and images that they view as threatening or dangerous. Note that the distinction between external and internal triggers is not always clear-cut. As you may have noticed, many of the examples of internal triggers you just read are anxiety-provoking only in the context of an external situation. For example, someone with social anxiety may be frightened by feeling shaky or sweaty, but only if there are other people around to notice. Similarly, someone with a fear of driving may fear being dizzy, but only when behind the wheel of a car. For some people, internal triggers may be anxiety-provoking only in the context of particular external triggers. For others, experiencing particular sensations or thoughts may be scary no matter where or when they occur.

Description of the Anxiety Disorders

As we've said, anxiety and fear are normal emotions that we all experience from time to time. Sometimes our anxiety and fear are realistic in the context, but often our reactions reflect unrealistic or exaggerated concerns. Almost everyone misinterprets events from time to time, so it's perfectly normal to experience unrealistic fear and anxiety on occasion. But if you experience exaggerated levels of anxiety and fear frequently, and the anxiety is causing problems in your day-to-day life, you may be experiencing an anxiety disorder. The American Psychiatric Association publishes a guide, the *Diagnostic and Statistical Manual of Mental Disorders* (DSM-IV-TR), for diagnosing psychological problems, including anxiety disorders. The current edition, DSM-IV-TR, lists more than 10 different anxiety disorders and provides specific criteria that health care professionals can use to decide whether an individual is suffering from one.

Table 1.1 provides a description of each anxiety disorder, as defined in DSM-IV-TR, along with a summary of the key features of each anxiety disorder. The process of diagnosing anxiety disorders or other problems is complex and requires extensive training. Sometimes even trained professionals can't agree on the best diagnosis to describe a particular person's problems. Although the information in this section will provide you with some clues regarding the types of problems you may be experiencing, it's best to be diagnosed by a professional who is experienced in assessing and diagnosing anxiety disorders.

table 1.1. **Summary of Key Features of the Anxiety Disorders**

Anxiety disorder	Key features
Panic disorder without agoraphobia	Recurrent, unexpected panic attacks without any obvious situational triggers
	Worry about having more panic attacks
	Concern about the consequences of panic attacks
	Changes in behavior as a result of the attacks
Panic disorder with agoraphobia	Same key features as above, with the addition of agoraphobia: a fear of situations in which escape might be difficult or help unavailable in the event of experiencing a panic attack or panic-like symptoms
	Typical situations feared by people with agoraphobia include crowds, being alone, driving, public transportation, and others
Agoraphobia without history of panic disorder	Fear of agoraphobic situations because of a concern about experiencing panic-like symptoms, but without a history of full-blown panic disorder
Social anxiety disorder	Fear of social or performance situations
	Excessive concern about being embarrassed or humiliated
Specific phobia	Fear of specific situations, such as animals, heights, storms, water, blood, injections, driving, flying, or enclosed places
Posttraumatic stress disorder	Occurs following a traumatic event during which the person responds with intense fear, helplessness, or horror
	Person reexperiences the event in memory, avoids reminders of the event, experiences numbing of his or her emotions, increased feelings of arousal, and a tendency to be on guard for possible danger
	Must be present for 1 month or longer
Acute stress disorder	Similar to posttraumatic stress disorder, but with a duration of 2 days to 4 weeks
Obsessive–compulsive disorder	Presence of obsessions: unwanted, repeated, intrusive thoughts, images, or urges that cause significant anxiety. Common obsessions involve contamination, doubting, and religious, sexual, or aggressive themes
	Presence of compulsions: behaviors designed to reduce anxiety or prevent bad things from happening. Common compulsions include checking, washing, counting, and repeating

(cont.)

table 1.1 *(cont.)*

Anxiety disorder	Key features
Generalized anxiety disorder	Excessive worry about many different things, lasting for at least 6 months, and accompanied by symptoms such as insomnia, fatigue, feeling keyed up and on edge, muscle tension, poor concentration, or irritability
Separation anxiety disorder	Extreme fear of being separated from key attachment figures, such as parents Usually diagnosed in childhood
Substance-induced anxiety disorder	Anxiety symptoms caused by the use of (or withdrawal from) a medication or other substance, such as cocaine, caffeine, or alcohol
Anxiety due to a general medical condition	Anxiety symptoms caused by a medical illness such as hyperthyroidism, heart disease, or diabetes
Anxiety disorder not otherwise specified	Significant anxiety symptoms that do not meet criteria for one of the other anxiety disorders

Panic Attack

A panic attack in itself is not actually an anxiety disorder, but it can be a feature of any of the anxiety disorders. Panic attacks also can occur in the context of other psychological problems. Moreover, many people without any particular psychological disorder experience panic attacks from time to time. The word *panic* comes from the name of the ancient Greek god *Pan,* who had the head and torso of a human and the hindquarters, legs, and horns of a goat, and who understandably inspired sudden fear among those who encountered him! Essentially, a panic attack is an episode of intense fear or discomfort that comes on quickly and includes a number of physical sensations or other symptoms. To be considered a full panic attack, the episode must include at least four of the following symptoms:

1. Racing or pounding heart
2. Sweating
3. Trembling or shaking
4. Shortness of breath or smothering sensations
5. Choking feelings
6. Chest pain or discomfort
7. Nausea or abdominal discomfort

8. Feelings of dizziness, lightheadedness, unsteadiness, or faintness
9. Feelings of unreality or detachment
10. Fear of losing control or going crazy
11. Fear of dying
12. Numbness or tingling sensations
13. Hot flushes or chills

According to the current DSM, panic attacks must peak within 10 minutes; many reach their high point within seconds. Panic attacks tend to last anywhere from a few minutes to an hour or so, though they often dissipate more quickly as soon as the person escapes from the threat. Often, panic attacks are triggered by some external situation—snakes, heights, driving, public speaking—but they can also be cued by an internal trigger, such as a feared sensation, thought, or image. Some panic attacks appear to occur out of the blue, without any obvious trigger or cue.

Panic Disorder with or without Agoraphobia

People with panic disorder experience panic attacks out of the blue, without any trigger or cause (at least not that they are aware of). In addition, perhaps more than any other anxiety disorder, panic disorder is associated with an extreme fear of itself—of having panic attacks and the physical sensations that occur during panic. People with panic disorder tend to worry about when their next attack will happen. They also worry about possible consequences of their attacks. For example, they may worry that they're having a heart attack or stroke, or that they may die, go crazy, lose control, vomit, have diarrhea, faint, or embarrass themselves in some way.

Because of these fears, people with panic disorder often alter their behavior to protect themselves from panicking or from suffering any dire consequences as a result of panic. For example, they may avoid situations where the attacks occur or they may rely on "safety" behaviors such as:

+ Carrying anti-anxiety medications in case a panic attack occurs
+ Always being accompanied by someone who makes them feel safe, like a spouse or a close friend
+ Carrying water to protect against a dry mouth
+ Frequently checking blood pressure or heart rate
+ Always staying near exits in public places
+ Driving with the window open for fear of not having enough fresh air

Most people with panic disorder also develop some degree of agoraphobia. *Agoraphobia* is a fear of being in places where escape might be difficult, or where help might not be available in the event of a panic attack or panic-like symptoms. The Greek word *agora* refers to the marketplace in ancient Greece. People with agoraphobia are often afraid of markets and other public places, as well as of many other situations that may arouse fear:

+ Driving (particularly in busy traffic, on highways, and on the inside lane)
+ Public transportation, including airplanes, buses, subways, boats, and trains
+ Crowded places, including sports venues, malls, supermarkets, museums, busy streets, theaters, classrooms, and the like
+ Situations from which escape is difficult, such as long lines, hair salons, dentist offices, business meetings, parties, and bridges
+ Enclosed places, such as small rooms, doctors' offices, tunnels, elevators, and parking garages
+ Being alone
+ Being far from home
+ Situations that trigger physical arousal symptoms, such as sex, exercise, and scary movies

People with panic disorder and agoraphobia tend to fear and avoid some of these situations. In severe cases, they may be frightened of all these situations and never leave their homes. The average person develops panic disorder in his or her 20s. This problem is considerably more prevalent among women than men. According to a recent study, about 4.7% of Americans suffer panic disorder with or without agoraphobia at some point in their lives; the prevalence is similar in other Western countries. Panic disorder often begins following a period of stress, such as unemployment, marital difficulties, having a new baby, or health problems.

Agoraphobia without History of Panic Disorder

Agoraphobia without a history of panic disorder occurs in only about 1.4% of people in the general population. People with agoraphobia might be afraid of experiencing panic-like symptoms, but they never experience full-blown panic attacks. Instead, they might experience attacks with fewer than the four symptoms needed to be called a panic attack.

Social Anxiety Disorder

Social anxiety disorder (SAD), also known as social phobia, is an extreme fear of situations in which a person might be observed, judged, or scrutinized. People with SAD are overly concerned about being embarrassed or humiliated, or of making a bad impression on others. Such a person tends to avoid situations involving direct interactions with others (interpersonal situations) and situations where he or she might be the center of attention (performance situations). Examples of *interpersonal situations* that are often feared by people with SAD include:

+ Initiating or maintaining conversations
+ Dating
+ Being assertive

+ Talking to people in authority
+ Parties, meetings, or other social gatherings

Examples of *performance situations* that are often feared by people with SAD include:

+ Speaking in front of groups
+ Eating or drinking in front of others
+ Writing in front of others
+ Being seen in public
+ Making mistakes in public
+ Working out in a gym with others around
+ Performing in public (for example, playing music, singing, acting)
+ Having one's picture taken

Some people with SAD fear only one situation (like public speaking) or a few situations, whereas others fear a wide range of social situations. But simply fearing these situations is not enough to warrant a diagnosis of SAD. After all, almost everyone feels anxious in social situations from time to time. Surveys have found that 40% of people report being chronically shy to the point of it being a problem, another 40% report having previously had problems with shyness, and a further 15% report being shy in some situations. In these surveys, only 5% of people reported never having difficulties with shyness!

In a study from our center conducted with college students, we found that experiencing anxiety symptoms in social situations was very common: almost everyone reported experiencing physical symptoms of anxiety at least occasionally in social situations. For example, more than three-quarters of people reported blushing on at least one occasion in a social situation. Other common experiences (reported by at least half of people) included heart palpitations, stammering, trouble expressing oneself, tension, wanting to escape, "butterflies" in the stomach, a lump in the throat, sweating, shaking, smiling or laughing inappropriately, and shaky voice.

To receive a diagnosis of SAD, an individual has to report excessive anxiety and fear in social situations that cause significant impairment or distress in his or her day-to-day life. In other words, the anxiety must interfere with your functioning at work or school, in relationships, or in other activities, or feel to you that it's a problem. SAD affects 12.1% of the general population at some point in their lives. It occurs about equally in men and women, though perhaps a bit more frequently in women. The average age of onset is in the teenage years, though it can begin in early childhood or in adulthood as well.

Specific Phobia

Specific phobia refers to an excessive or unrealistic fear of a specific object or situation. Like SAD, specific phobias are not diagnosed unless the fear interferes with the individual's life or is experienced as being a problem. For example, if you're terrified of snakes but you live in an area where there aren't any snakes, you would not be considered to have a phobia. DSM-IV-TR includes four main types of specific phobias, and a fifth to capture those phobias that are not included in the other four:

1. *Animal type*: These can include fears of any animal or insect. Some of the more common ones are dogs, cats, mice, spiders, snakes, bugs, moths, cockroaches, birds, and lizards.
2. *Natural environment type*: These include fears of heights, water, storms, and the dark.
3. *Blood/injection/injury type*: These include fears of the sight of blood, watching surgery, receiving a shot, having blood tests, having dental procedures, and related problems. This is the only type of anxiety problem that is often associated with fainting. (About 70% of people with blood phobias and just over half of people with needle phobias report having fainted in the situation.) The fainting is related to a sudden drop in heart rate and blood pressure in the feared situation. (With other fears, heart rate and blood pressure tend to *increase* in the situation.)
4. *Situational type*: These include specific fears of flying, driving, enclosed places, and related situations.
5. *Other type*: These include other specific phobias, for example, fear of clowns.

According to recent estimates, about 12.5% of the general population have a specific phobia at some point in their lives. Of these, the most common are animal phobias (especially fears of creepy-crawly animals like spiders and snakes) and height phobias, but most of the phobia types in the list are fairly common. Some specific phobias (for example, animal phobias and storm phobias) are much more common in women than in men, whereas others (for example, blood/injection/injury phobias) are about equally common in men and women.

Animal phobias tend to begin in childhood, whereas situational phobias are more likely to begin in early adulthood. Blood/injection/injury phobias and natural environment phobias tend to begin in childhood or in the teens.

Posttraumatic Stress Disorder and Acute Stress Disorder

Posttraumatic stress disorder (PTSD) is an anxiety disorder that begins following a serious trauma in which a person's life or physical well-being is threatened. Examples of PTSD traumas include:

+ Sexual abuse, assault, or rape
+ Physical abuse or assault
+ Being a victim of armed robbery
+ Serious accidents at work, at home, while driving, or elsewhere
+ Combat

✦ Seeing someone get killed or badly hurt

✦ Surviving a fire, earthquake, serious storm, or other disaster

During the trauma, the individual's response is one of fear, helplessness, or horror. In addition, people with PTSD develop symptoms from each of three main clusters or groups. The first includes symptoms involving mentally reexperiencing the trauma. This includes repeated disturbing memories of the trauma, nightmares about it, flashbacks in which it feels as though the trauma is happening again, and becoming very upset and anxious upon being reminded of the trauma.

The second cluster includes symptoms involving avoidance of situations that remind the person of the trauma and a general numbing of the person's emotions. Examples include a tendency to avoid thoughts, feelings, conversations, activities, people, and places that remind the individual of the trauma; an inability to remember aspects of the trauma; feeling detached or different from others; a lack of interest in important activities; an inability to experience happy feelings; and a sense that one's life may be cut short.

The third cluster includes symptoms involving a heightened awareness of one's surroundings and increased arousal. These include such things as difficulty sleeping, anger problems, trouble concentrating, always having to be on guard for possible danger, and being startled easily.

A diagnosis of PTSD requires that the symptoms be present for at least 1 month. In contrast, a diagnosis of acute stress disorder requires many of the same symptoms, but for a shorter period (lasting anywhere from 2 days to 4 weeks). In many cases, people may receive a diagnosis of acute stress disorder after a trauma, and then see it changed to PTSD if the problems continue after a month.

The prevalence of PTSD in the general population is about 6.8%. The age of onset varies, depending on when the trauma occurred. Most people who experience a trauma don't develop PTSD. They may experience significant PTSD-like symptoms in the early days following a trauma, but for most the symptoms will improve over time. And some people develop problems other than PTSD following a trauma. A sexual assault may lead to PTSD in some people, for example, and in others to problems with depression, substance use, or relationships.

Obsessive–Compulsive Disorder

Obsessions are irrational thoughts, images, or urges that a person has frequently and that are experienced as intrusive, inappropriate, upsetting, distressing, or frightening. Table 1.2 shows some examples of common obsessions.

Compulsions are behaviors that people use to reduce the anxiety caused by their obsessions. These activities may follow a rigid, self-imposed set of rules that the person believes will prevent bad things from happening. Whereas obsessions tend to make people more uncomfortable and anxious, compulsions reduce their anxiety and discomfort. Examples of common compulsions are described in Table 1.3, along with what percentage of people with obsessive–compulsive disorder (OCD) in our center report each type of compulsion. Although most people with OCD have both obsessions and compulsions, it is possible to have OCD with just obsessions or just compulsions.

Many people have doubts about whether they locked the door, concerns about contamination, even occasional thoughts about hurting a loved one. (In a recent study, consumers were less likely to purchase a product in a store if they believed it had been touched by someone else, even if they didn't actually see another person touch the product.) Does this mean that everyone has OCD? Not at all. A diagnosis of OCD

table 1.2. **Common Types of Obsessions and the Percentage of People with OCD Who Report Experiencing Each Type**

Type of obsession	Examples	Percent
Aggressive obsessions	Unrealistic fears of hurting a loved one (for example, stabbing, strangling, or pushing him or her into traffic)	68.7%
Contamination obsessions	Fear of coming into contact with germs, toxins, detergents, chemicals, diseases, and the like	57.7%
Symmetry and exactness obsessions	Need to have things just right (for example, books in order on the bookshelf, pillows all lined up on the sofa, and so on)	53.2%
Somatic obsessions (obsessions related to the body)	Repeated thoughts about a body part or function (for example, being excessively focused on one's blinking, being convinced that one is giving off a particular odor, being fearful of having one body part touch another, and the like)	34.1%
Hoarding and saving-related obsessions	Urges to keep useless objects or to collect things excessively	30.2%
Religious obsessions	Intrusive thoughts or images of Satan or other "forbidden" religious symbols, repeated blasphemous thoughts	24.2%
Sexual obsessions	Unrealistic sexual thoughts that the person finds disturbing (for example, worrying about being gay despite all evidence saying otherwise, irrational worries about being a pedophile)	19.8%
Miscellaneous obsessions	Other repetitive thoughts that an individual finds disturbing or frightening	55.5%

Based on data reported by Antony, M. M., Downie, F., & Swinson, R. P. (1998). Diagnostic issues and epidemiology in obsessive compulsive disorder. In R. P. Swinson, M. M. Antony, S. Rachman, & M. A. Richter (Eds.), *Obsessive–compulsive disorder: Theory, research, and treatment* (pp. 3–32). New York: Guilford Press.

table 1.3. **Common Types of Compulsions and the Percentage of People with OCD Who Report Experiencing Each Type**

Type of compulsion	Examples	Percent
Checking	Checking to see that the stove is off, the doors are locked, work is completed properly, and so on	80.7%
Washing and cleaning	Excessive hand washing (for example, hundreds of times each day), excessive house cleaning, repeatedly washing the same clothes in the laundry, and the like	63.7%
Repeating	Repeating actions, words, prayers, and so on, over and over again—for example, opening and closing doors repeatedly until it "feels" right	55.5%
Ordering or arranging	Spending hours lining objects up on various surfaces according to particular rules; arranging items in the kitchen cabinets according to size	40.1%
Counting	Counting tiles on the ceiling; counting blinks; counting words; doing things in even numbers; and the like	35.2%
Hoarding	Buying the same T-shirt in every color; buying 30 watchbands because they are on sale; refusing to discard any receipts in case they will be needed in the future	28.0%
Miscellaneous compulsions	Other repeated behaviors (for example, touching objects; adding numbers and letters on license plates; and so on)	59.3%

Based on data reported by Antony, M. M., Downie, F., & Swinson, R. P. (1998). Diagnostic issues and epidemiology in obsessive compulsive disorder. In R. P. Swinson, M. M. Antony, S. Rachman, & M. A. Richter (Eds.), *Obsessive–compulsive disorder: Theory, research, and treatment* (pp. 3–32). New York: Guilford Press.

requires that the obsessions and compulsions lead to significant interference, that they bother the person, or that they take up at least an hour every day. One study found that 1.6% of people in the general population have symptoms meeting the official criteria for OCD. The disorder is about equally common among adult men and women, though perhaps a bit more common in women. In children, however, OCD appears to be more common in boys than in girls.

Generalized Anxiety Disorder

People with generalized anxiety disorder (GAD) are worriers. They worry about a wide range of topics: work, school, their family, their health, money, the world, and minor matters that arise from day to day. What distinguishes the kind of worrying that would lead a person to be diagnosed with GAD?

First, it needs to have been a long-standing problem—for at least 6 months. Many people with GAD describe themselves as having been worriers for as long as they can remember. Second, the worry must be about many different things. If a person only worries about work, that's not GAD. Third, the worry must be excessive, out of proportion to the actual situation. Worrying about your elderly father who is being treated for a serious illness would not be excessive worry. Fourth, the excessive worry must be frequent—occurring on most days. To receive a diagnosis of GAD, the individual must also experience at least three of the following symptoms on an ongoing basis: feeling restless, keyed up, or on edge; poor concentration; muscle tension; sleep problems; fatigue; and difficulties with irritability or anger.

GAD affects about 5.7% of the population. It occurs more often in women than men, and it often occurs along with problems like depression and other anxiety disorders.

Separation Anxiety Disorder

The core feature of separation anxiety disorder is a fear of separation from home or from key figures in a person's life. This disorder is usually diagnosed in children, though it can persist into adulthood. Examples of features often associated with this problem include:

+ Excessive anxiety when separated from home or from major "attachment figures" such as parents or other close relatives
+ Worry about losing, or harm coming to, close attachment figures
+ Worry that some negative event (for example, being kidnapped) will lead to separation from key attachment figures
+ Refusal to go to school or elsewhere due to a fear of separation
+ An excessive fear of being alone, even at home
+ A fear of going to sleep without key attachment figures close by (for example, a fear of sleeping away from home without one's parents)
+ Repeated nightmares involving themes of separation
+ Uncomfortable physical symptoms whenever separation occurs or is expected

Separation anxiety disorder always begins in childhood (that's one of the official diagnostic criteria). Recent estimates suggest that 5.2% of the general population has suffered from this problem at some point in their lives. Many of these individuals have either outgrown the problem by adulthood or seen it develop into a different anxiety-based problem over time. For example, some researchers have suggested that separation anxiety disorder in children may develop into panic disorder and agoraphobia in some adults, in part because these two conditions share many features (fear of being alone, uncomfortable physical sensations upon separation, and so on). Very little is known about the nature and treatment of separation anxiety disorder in adults, as most of the research on this problem has been based on children.

Substance-Induced Anxiety Disorder and Anxiety Due to a General Medical Condition

Before a diagnosis of anxiety disorder can be made, the direct effects of a substance or of a medical illness must be ruled out. Exceptions to this rule are anxiety disorders that are caused by just these things.

In the case of substance-induced anxiety disorder, the anxiety symptoms are entirely due to a medication, an illegal drug, or some other substance. A person might have panic attacks, for example, after drinking too much coffee, using cocaine, taking medications with stimulant properties, or withdrawing from alcohol use. If the anxiety symptoms persist even after the substance use has stopped (or the withdrawal phase is complete), then a different anxiety disorder diagnosis should be considered. The person who drinks 10 cups of coffee daily who continues to have panic attacks after cutting out coffee might receive a diagnosis of panic disorder.

In anxiety disorder due to a general medical condition, the anxiety symptoms are due entirely to a medical illness. OCD symptoms might be triggered by a brain tumor, for instance, or panic attacks might be triggered by an overactive thyroid. If the anxiety continues after the medical illness has been successfully treated, then diagnosis of another anxiety disorder may be appropriate.

Note that medical problems can sometimes make an underlying anxiety disorder worse, though not be completely responsible for it. For example, someone with panic disorder who also has asthma may experience more severe panic attacks. Such cases would not be diagnosed in this category.

Anxiety Disorder Not Otherwise Specified

Anxiety disorder not otherwise specified (ADNOS) is a category reserved for anxiety problems that don't fit neatly into one of the other main categories. For example, if someone was experiencing PTSD symptoms but didn't have enough symptoms to warrant a diagnosis of PTSD, a diagnosis of ADNOS might be assigned, assuming the problem was severe enough to warrant a diagnosis at all.

Other Anxiety-Related Problems

Although DSM-IV-TR lists 10 official anxiety disorders, there are a number of other problems that have anxiety as a core feature. The strategies in this book are often helpful for some of these other anxiety-related problems too.

Hypochondriasis (Health Anxiety)

Hypochondriasis is a problem in which people are overly concerned about the possibility of having a serious disease, based on a tendency to misinterpret normal bodily symptoms. A person with hypochondriasis may misinterpret a spot on the skin as a sign of skin cancer or a headache as a sign of a brain tumor. People with hypochondriasis visit their doctors frequently to check out various physical symptoms, but the reassurance they receive from the doctor rarely lasts very long. Hypochondriasis shares features with panic disorder (for example, a fear of bodily sensations), as well as with GAD (for example, a tendency to worry about health) and OCD (for example, a tendency to check excessively and ask for reassurance).

Obsessive–Compulsive Personality Disorder

Obsessive–compulsive personality disorder (OCPD) is a problem in which people are preoccupied with orderliness, perfectionism, and a need to be in control. People with OCPD tend to be overly concerned with details, rules, schedules, lists, and organization to the point that it is difficult for them to complete tasks; the original purpose of the activity often gets buried in a mountain of detail. People with OCPD often have difficulty delegating tasks to other people and are frequently described as overconscientious and rigid. OCPD is often driven by anxiety-related beliefs that giving up control will lead to chaos in one's life. It can be difficult to distinguish it from some types of OCD; indeed, the two problems often co-occur.

Body Dysmorphic Disorder (Imagined Ugliness)

In body dysmorphic disorder (BDD), the core feature is an imagined defect in appearance. A person with a BDD may be preoccupied with thoughts of having a big nose, an asymmetrical face, or funny-shaped legs, which others don't see. People with BDD often think constantly about their "defect," taking great pains to hide it from others and checking frequently to make sure it stays hidden. BDD shares features with other anxiety disorders such as social anxiety disorder (for example, a fear of being observed by others) and OCD (for example, excessive checking).

Fear of Death

It's normal to fear death, and most of us do. As with any anxiety problem, it's only a concern if the fear causes you significant distress or interferes with your life. Fear of death is often a feature of another anxiety disorder. For example, people with panic disorder may worry about dying during a panic attack, people with GAD may worry about dying in general, and some people with OCD may ruminate about dying after coming into contact with some sort of contaminant that they view as dangerous. But excessive fear of death can also occur in the absence of another anxiety disorder.

Test Anxiety

Anxiety about exams or tests is another problem for which the strategies in this book may be useful. As with death anxiety, it may be a feature of another anxiety disorder. People with panic disorder may be nervous about exams, fearing they may panic and be unable to leave the exam room. People with social anxiety may worry about being judged or evaluated if they do poorly on an exam and will be particularly anxious about oral exams and presentations. People with OCD may fear tests because of a concern about making mistakes and the need to check their work over and over. People with GAD may worry about tests and exams because they worry about almost everything. Test anxiety can also exist in the absence of any other specific anxiety-based problem. For example, people with poor study skills who tend to get low grades may have realistic anxiety about tests.

Distinguishing between Anxiety-Based Problems

For a number of reasons, it's often difficult for psychologists and psychiatrists to figure out which anxiety disorder a person has. People's problems don't always fit into neat categories. An anxiety problem may share features of several anxiety disorders while not meeting all the criteria of any specific one. And the features of the various anxiety problems overlap. For example, a fear of flying can occur for many reasons: in panic disorder with agoraphobia, a person may fear panicking and not being able to escape from the plane; in a specific phobia, a person may fear a plane crash; in social phobia, a person may fear having to talk to the person in the next seat.

Similarly, anxiety in social situations can occur across most of the anxiety disorders. People with social anxiety may be fearful of looking foolish in front of other people; people with OCD may be anxious that others will notice them repeatedly counting things or washing their hands.

Although it is useful to understand the similarities and differences between the various anxiety disorders, you don't have to know with absolute certainty which anxiety disorder you're experiencing in order to benefit from this book. As you will discover, similar treatment strategies have been found to be useful for different anxiety disorders. The methods described in this book are designed to be used for symptoms of anxiety and fear regardless of the particular anxiety disorder or disorders. This is important because for many people anxiety disorders occur in clusters. Most people with one anxiety disorder also experience features of other anxiety disorders, as well as different problems, like depression.

Causes of Anxiety and the Anxiety Disorders

Anxiety and anxiety disorders do not spring from any one cause. Rather, many different variables seem to influence who develops an anxiety problem and what sort of anxiety problem he or she develops: biological factors, psychological factors, lifestyle factors, and societal and cultural factors, among others. Of course, it's often impossible to know which factors are responsible for any one person's anxiety problem. Fortunately, we don't need to understand the cause of a person's anxiety to develop an effective treatment plan.

Biological Influences

Our knowledge about the effects of biology on the development and course of anxiety-based problems comes from research studies on genetics, brain chemistry, and specific areas of the brain that may be involved in anxiety.

Inheriting Anxiety

We inherit the tendency to be anxious or tense. Anxiety disorders run in families. Our genetic makeup seems to influence the transmission of anxiety-based problems from one generation to the next. Unlike traits like eye color (for which the influence of genetics is straightforward and well understood), however, the influence of genetics on the development of anxiety disorders is complex and probably involves many different genes. Also, genetics is only one of many different factors that contribute to the development of anxiety disorders.

One of the challenges in trying to sort out the extent to which an anxiety disorder is inherited involves separating out the effects of genetics and environment. Family members share their genes, but they also share experiences. For example, brothers and sisters live in the same homes, often go to the same schools, grow up during the same period, and have the same parents. To tease out the effects of genetics and environment, scientists often study large groups of twins. If an anxiety problem was based entirely on genetics, the identical twin of a person suffering from an anxiety disorder should have the same anxiety disorder. If the transmission of anxiety disorders across generations were based completely on a shared environment, one might expect the frequency of anxiety disorders to be about the same in identical twins and fraternal twins of individuals with anxiety disorders, assuming they grew up in similar environments.

Neither of these scenarios seems to be the case. Having an identical twin with an anxiety-based problem does not guarantee that a person will develop an anxiety disorder. However, the rate of anxiety disorders does tend to be higher between identical twins than between fraternal twins. Some studies show a stronger influence of genetics than do others, and studies often disagree about which anxiety disorders are most strongly influenced by genetics. Nevertheless, taking into account the pattern of findings across twin studies as well as other types of genetic research, there is little doubt that genetics influences the development of anxiety.

Brain Chemistry

The brain is like a chemical factory. Information is transmitted from one nerve cell to the next by chemical messengers called *neurotransmitters*. Each nerve cell (or neuron) releases small amounts of neurotransmitter, some of which triggers a reaction in the next neuron and some of which is reabsorbed by the original neuron (in a process known as *reuptake*). The effects of this process on our body depend on the type of neurotransmitter released, the amount that is produced, the amount that is reabsorbed, the sensitivity of the receptors on the receiving neuron, and the location in the brain where the process is occurring. Examples of neurotransmitters that are believed to play a role in anxiety disorders include serotonin, norepinephrine, and gamma-aminobutyric acid (GABA).

It's believed, for example, that serotonin is involved in OCD. Medications that increase levels of serotonin in the brain are often useful for treating OCD. These include the selective serotonin reuptake inhibitors (SSRIs), such as paroxetine (Paxil) and fluoxetine (Prozac), as well as certain other medications. In contrast, medications that primarily influence other neurotransmitters are not particularly effective for treating OCD. In the case of panic disorder, there is evidence that substances that increase norepinephrine levels in the brain (for example, injections of sodium lactate) can trigger panic attacks, whereas medications that block the reuptake of norepinephrine (for example, imipramine or Tofranil) are often useful for treating panic disorder. The evidence also indicates that other neurotransmitters, such as serotonin, play a role in panic disorder.

Understanding the role of neurotransmitters in anxiety disorders has been helpful for developing new medications for anxiety. But the relationship between neurotransmitters and anxiety disorders is complex and still poorly understood. We can't tell from an individual's levels of any particular neurotransmitter whether he or she is likely to have an anxiety problem. Nor can we test for a specific chemical imbalance and use that information to predict a person's likelihood of success with a particular medication. What we do know is (1) that when we average across many different people, medications that affect neurotransmitters often reduce anxiety; and (2) that there are differences in how neurotransmitters function among groups of people *with* anxiety disorders and people *without* anxiety disorders.

Brain Activity

Advances in technology have provided scientists with exciting new tools to measure brain activity. For example, positron emission tomography (PET) and functional magnetic resonance imaging (fMRI) are imaging techniques that allow researchers to measure patterns of blood flow in the brain, just as X-rays can be used to provide images of bones. These imaging techniques can identify areas of the brain that are more or less active in particular anxiety disorders. People with OCD have been found to have distinct patterns of brain activity, for example, and there may even be differences in brain function among people with specific subtypes of OCD (for example, people who wash versus people who check).

But findings from brain imaging studies are often not consistent. Also, it's difficult to conclude much about the cause of an anxiety disorder based on findings from brain imaging studies because an area of increased activity in the brain may indicate something about the *cause* of a person's anxiety disorder or it may simply be an *effect* of having the anxiety disorder.

Psychological Influences

Although biological research has contributed greatly to our understanding of anxiety, we also possess a wealth of knowledge about the influence of psychological factors.

Some of the most important psychological factors known to underlie anxiety disorders include the role of learning and experience, the role of one's thoughts and beliefs, and the role of one's behaviors.

Learning and Experiences

Think about some of the most memorable experiences you've had, both good and bad. These may include the breakup of a relationship, meeting a new friend, having an accident, the death of a loved one, a fantastic course that you took in school, or even a movie that changed you in some way. We are all shaped by our histories. Psychologist Stanley Rachman proposed three types of experiences through which we learn to experience anxiety and fear in response to particular objects and situations.

One is *direct experience.* That's when we learn to fear an object or situation through some sort of direct negative or traumatic experience. Some examples include:

- Learning to fear dogs after being bitten by a dog
- Learning to fear flying after enduring a very turbulent flight
- Learning to fear driving after a car accident
- Developing a fear of public speaking after being teased following a presentation
- Learning to fear eating certain foods after suffering a bout of food poisoning

Considerable evidence indicates that negative experiences can influence fear and anxiety. In the case of PTSD and acute stress disorder, a negative experience is always the trigger. But even in the other anxiety disorders, people often report a history of one or more traumatic experiences that either initially caused the anxiety or led to a worsening of it.

Rachman's second pathway to developing fear is learning through *observation.* This happens when you learn to fear a situation by watching somebody else have a negative experience or behave fearfully in a situation. This may explain how an individual's environment can contribute to the transmission of anxiety from generation to generation. For example, a child who grows up with a parent who is terrified of driving may develop his or her own fear of getting behind the wheel. When a situation is unfamiliar, children often take their cues from their parents before deciding whether a situation is safe or dangerous. Watching a trusted parent panic whenever he or she encounters a particular object or situation may teach a child to fear that object or situation as well.

Rachman's third pathway to developing fear and anxiety involves learning through *information or instruction*—in other words, learning to fear situations via material you encounter through conversations, reading, watching television, and other sources of information. For example, a small boy may learn to fear germs and disease if his parents frequently warn him about the dangers of coming into contact with germs. An important route of informational learning is the influence of the news media on various fears. After the 9/11 terrorist attacks, many people were reluctant to fly. Several airlines around the world even ended up declaring bankruptcy; in the United States alone more than 100,000 people lost their jobs in various airline-related businesses. People's fear of flying was probably triggered by vivid images in the media. Of course, statistically speaking, flying continues to be a very safe way of traveling.

Although these three pathways explain the occurrence of fear in some cases, they don't fully explain the relationship between learning and fear. For example, many people develop problems with fear and anxiety without ever having a negative experience, watching somebody else be afraid, or hearing about the dangers associated with a situation they fear. For some people, fears seem to begin out of the blue. And many people who have these negative experiences do not develop fears. So although these pathways may contribute to the development of fears, they don't really explain why some people develop significant fears following these experiences and others don't. It's likely that other factors (such as genetic vulnerabilities, personality styles, beliefs about the experience, behavior following the experience, and the like) also play a role.

Thinking and Anxiety

Anxiety disorders are associated with negative patterns of thinking, and having negative thoughts can contribute to anxiety and fear. One of the main differences between someone who fears driving and someone who doesn't is that the former believes that the situation is threatening or dangerous. In fact, many experts hold that in order to experience fear in a situation, the situation must be interpreted as dangerous in some way. Table 1.4 includes examples of thoughts, beliefs, predictions, and assumptions that may contribute to fear and anxiety in particular anxiety disorders.

Behavior and Anxiety

How people behave in response to their anxiety has a big effect on whether they manage to overcome it. Two types of behavior seem to be the most problematic. The first is *avoidance*. It's natural to want to avoid a situation that triggers anxiety or fear, but avoidance helps keep the anxiety alive over time. Avoiding the feared situation means you'll probably never learn that it is indeed safe, and your anxiety may never have a chance to decrease. Although avoidance helps keep your anxiety under control in the short term, it has the exact opposite effect over the long term.

Safety behaviors are a second strategy that people often use to reduce their anxiety in the short term, but, as with avoidance, they actually help the anxiety along. In fact, safety behaviors can be thought of as a more subtle form of avoidance. The compulsions that are often part of OCD can also be viewed as extreme safety behaviors. Some examples of safety behaviors include:

- ✦ Repetitive hand washing to avoid getting sick
- ✦ Using distraction to prevent panic attacks
- ✦ Wearing a turtleneck sweater or extra makeup to hide blushing
- ✦ Wearing gloves to avoid coming into contact with germs
- ✦ Carrying a gun or knife to protect against possible attackers

table 1.4. **Common Beliefs Associated with Various Anxiety Disorders**

Anxiety disorder	Examples of common beliefs
Panic disorder with or without agoraphobia	"A racing heart is a sign that I may be having a heart attack." "It would be terrible to panic in a movie theater." "I could faint during a panic attack." "A feeling of unreality is a sign that I may be losing control or going crazy."
Specific phobias	"The dog will attack me." "The plane will crash." "I will run out of air on the elevator." "If I get dizzy, I will fall from a high place."
Social anxiety disorder	"I will make a fool of myself during the presentation." "People find me boring." "My boss will think I'm incompetent." "Nobody would ever want to date me."
Obsessive–compulsive disorder	"If I don't wash my hands frequently, I'll get sick." "If I think about hurting a loved one, it means that I'm more likely to do it." "I need to check my work over and over because it would be a disaster to make a mistake." "I can't throw anything away in case I may need it later."
Generalized anxiety disorder	"My husband is probably late because he's been in a car accident." "It would be terrible to be late for an appointment." "Worrying helps to prepare me for bad things that may happen." "I need to be the perfect parent."
Posttraumatic stress disorder (following a sexual assault)	"If I go out alone, I will be attacked." "I should have been able to prevent the rape." "All men are potentially dangerous." "People will think worse of me if they know that I was raped."

+ Always being accompanied by someone else in public places to feel more comfortable
+ Carrying anti-anxiety medication just in case the anxiety gets out of control

Societal and Cultural Influences

Anxiety disorders occur throughout the world and across cultures, but culture can influence the *content* of a person's anxiety. Many of the anxiety syndromes described in this chapter may not occur as commonly in non-Western cultures, at least not in the same form. And non-Western cultures often experience anxiety problems that would be considered unusual in the West. For example, *koro*, an anxiety disorder that occurs in some East Asian cultures, is associated with sudden and intense anxiety that the penis (or in females, the vulva and nipples) will recede into the body, possibly causing death. *Taijin kyofusho*, a phobia that occurs in Japan, is an intense fear that an aspect of one's body may be unpleasant, embarrassing, or offensive to others.

Even in the Western world the content of a person's fear may be influenced by the individual's job, religion, or other aspects of the surrounding culture or environment. For example, people with OCD who are very religious are more likely to have obsessions with religious themes than obsessions focused on things like contamination.

Cultural factors may also help explain why some fears are more common in women than in men. In Western cultures it is much more acceptable for women to express fear and anxiety than it is for men. Men may choose to hide their feelings of anxiety, or to mask them by drinking or by responding to perceived threats with an aggressive or angry response.

As discussed earlier, the news media may also have an impact on what situations we fear. People often fear the sorts of threats that the media tell us to fear: terrorism, shark attacks, tainted food, plane crashes, murder, and mysterious diseases like severe acute respiratory syndrome (SARS), bird flu, and anthrax poisoning. Although these threats harm a very small minority of the population, they tend to arouse greater fear than more dangerous (and more subtle) threats such as smoking, alcohol abuse, and obesity.

Overview of Effective Treatments

With all the complications of their many causes and faces, the good news is that anxiety and anxiety disorders are among the most treatable of psychological problems. This section provides a brief overview of the treatments that will be discussed in detail throughout this book. You will notice that certain treatments are not discussed in this section—for example, hypnosis and traditional psychotherapies. That's because they haven't been studied extensively for the treatment of anxiety disorders, so their effects remain unproven.

Medication and Biological Treatments

Two major classes of medications have been found to be effective for anxiety disorders. One includes *antidepressants* such as paroxetine (Paxil), venlaxafine (Effexor), and others. Don't be misled by the name "antidepressants": they are called antidepressants because they were originally developed for treating depression. However, these medications are very effective for treating most anxiety disorders, even when an individual is not depressed. In fact, they're used for lots of problems other than depression—anxiety disorders, as well as eating disorders and pain management, among other conditions.

The *anxiolytics* or *anti-anxiety medications* are the other type of drug that proves useful for treating anxiety problems. These include benzodiazepines, such as diazepam (Valium) and lorazepam (Ativan), as well as other drugs. Generally, these medications are prescribed by family physicians, psychiatrists, or other physicians, though some states also allow other professionals to prescribe them.

Certain over-the-counter herbal products may also be useful for treating anxiety-based problems, though in many cases claims regarding these products have not been backed up by adequate research. Medications and herbal remedies are discussed in detail in Chapter 10.

Cognitive Approaches

As discussed earlier, anxiety is often influenced by the sorts of thoughts, predictions, and assumptions we hold about the situation we fear. Cognitive approaches to treating anxiety involve learning to identify the sorts of thoughts that contribute to your anxiety and finding ways to replace these thoughts with more realistic and balanced predictions and assumptions. The first step in this process is acknowledging that your anxious predictions are merely guesses about what might happen. Once you recognize that your anxious beliefs may not be true, the next step is to consider other ways of viewing the situation, followed by a thorough examination of the evidence. Often this process leads to a shift in thinking, and ultimately to a shift in anxious feelings. Cognitive strategies for changing your anxiety are discussed in Chapter 4.

Behavioral Approaches

Behavioral strategies focus on changing behaviors that contribute to your problems with anxiety. Primarily, these involve breaking the habits of avoidance, employing safety behaviors, and following compulsive rituals. By learning to confront the situations you fear instead of avoiding and protecting yourself from "dangers" that in reality are minimal or nonexistent, you will learn that your anxious predictions don't come true. Don't be overwhelmed by the thought of exposure to feared situations. As you will see, exposure is conducted gradually, so the fear you experience will be manageable.

And it will be well worth it. Exposure is one of the most powerful ways of overcoming fear, and the gains from exposure tend to be very long lasting. In addition to situational exposure (discussed in Chapters 5 and 6), this book also includes discussion of how exposure can be used to overcome a fear of thoughts, memories, and images (Chapter 7), and how exposure to physical symptoms can be used to overcome a fear of physical sensations, like a racing heart or dizziness (Chapter 8).

Relaxation-, Meditation-, and Acceptance-Based Treatments

Relaxation-based strategies have been used for decades to treat anxiety-related concerns. These include exercises involving tensing and relaxing the muscles of the body, slowing down one's breathing, and imagining relaxing scenes, as described in Chapter 9. Although relaxation training is somewhat useful for a range of anxiety problems, for most anxiety disorders this approach has not been found to be as effective as treatments involving exposure or cognitive strategies. One exception is GAD, for which relaxation is among the most effective methods. People with other types of anxiety, especially anxiety focused on specific situations (for example, social anxiety) would be advised to focus on some of the other strategies.

Another technique is meditation. Since anxiety is an unpleasant emotion, it's natural to want to do whatever we can to reduce it. But efforts to fight anxiety, to distract ourselves from it, or to "make" it go away often have the opposite effect. Meditation is not new—it has been used for thousands of years to deal with feelings of anxiety and stress. Only recently, though, have scientists begun to study its effectiveness in treating anxiety disorders. So far, the news is promising. Preliminary evidence supports the use of meditation-based strategies, at least for generalized anxiety and worry.

Related therapies focus on teaching people to accept their anxious feelings rather than fight them. An example is a treatment called *acceptance and commitment therapy*. It's too early to know whether meditation- and acceptance-based strategies are as powerful as the better established cognitive and exposure-based strategies, but the early evidence suggests that these treatments are likely to be useful. Meditation- and acceptance-based strategies are discussed in Chapter 9. There is also much debate among experts about whether the new acceptance-based treatments are actually different from more established psychological treatments. As you will see throughout this book, cognitive- and exposure-based strategies also encourage people to accept their anxious feelings rather than fight them.

Lifestyle Interventions

Chapter 11 discusses the role of lifestyle and health habits in anxiety. For example, people with anxiety disorders are more likely to smoke than people without anxiety disorders. Nicotine is a stimulant that can make anxiety symptoms worse. Drinking too much coffee or other caffeinated beverages can also increase anxiety levels, as can certain medications and illegal drugs (especially stimulants), and withdrawal from alcohol. Maintaining good nutrition, regular exercise, and good sleep habits are likely to help you in managing your anxiety.

Conclusion

Anxiety and fear are perfectly normal emotions designed to protect us from potential danger. Perceived threats that trigger anxiety can include external situations or objects, or internal experiences, such as certain physical sensations and thoughts. The sensations that occur during a panic attack can be particularly frightening. The strategies discussed in this book are likely to be useful for a wide range of problems, including panic disorder with or without agoraphobia, social anxiety disorder, specific phobia, PTSD, OCD, GAD, separation anxiety, health anxiety, and other anxiety-based problems.

Anxiety disorders develop through a complex interaction of biological, psychological, and social factors. Genetics play a role in the development of anxiety, and specific patterns of brain chemistry are associated with anxiety-based problems. The development and maintenance of anxiety are also associated with certain types of experiences, a tendency to think in anxious ways, and a tendency to rely on avoidance and safety behaviors to cope with anxiety and fear. You can overcome anxiety by changing your patterns of thinking and behavior that have been helping it to flourish. Confronting a feared situation through exposure therapy is one of the most powerful ways of reducing its hold on you. Learning to think in a less anxious way about frightening situations is also useful for reducing anxiety, as are relaxation-, meditation-, and acceptance-based strategies. Finally, a variety of medications have been found useful for treating most of the anxiety disorders. Psychological treatments and medications may be used separately or in combination. Regardless of how you choose to work on your anxiety, however, the first step is the most important one in your journey toward ridding yourself of your excessive anxiety and fear. And starting this book is an excellent first step!

2

Getting to Know Your Anxiety

Before beginning to work on freeing yourself from your anxiety problem, you need to understand it better. In Chapter 1, you learned all about anxiety in general. In this chapter, you'll learn about *your own* anxiety. Developing a treatment plan must take into account the specific situations and experiences that trigger your anxiety, as well as the ways in which you personally respond to these triggers. This chapter shows you how to conduct a self-assessment that is similar to the kind of thing a professional therapist might do with you during a first visit. This is a critical first step because the specific treatment strategies in this workbook that you will end up using will depend on what you find out here. In this chapter, you will identify:

+ Situations and objects that trigger your fear
+ The variables that affect your fear
+ Physical sensations associated with your anxiety and fear
+ Anxiety-provoking thoughts and beliefs
+ The ways in which you avoid external fear triggers
+ Safety behaviors that you use to protect yourself from possible danger
+ The extent to which you fear and avoid certain internal experiences, such as thoughts, images, or physical sensations
+ Other associated problems, like depression or conflict in your relationships

What Situations and Objects Trigger Your Fear and Anxiety?

The situations and objects that trigger anxiety and fear differ from person to person. Table 2.1 includes some examples of situational triggers for various types of anxiety problems. After reviewing it, generate a list of situations and objects that trigger your fear and record them in Form 2.1. You may include examples from the table, but try to come up with some others too. If you have more than one anxiety problem (for example, you might have panic disorder, social anxiety, and a fear of dogs), list your triggers for

table 2.1. **Common Situational Triggers for Various Anxiety Problems**

Anxiety problem	Common situational triggers
Panic disorder and agoraphobia	*Situations that trigger fear of having a panic attack* Being alone Being away from home Transportation: cars, planes, buses, trains, subways Crowded places: restaurants, supermarkets, malls, theaters, arenas, busy streets Enclosed places: small rooms, tunnels, elevators Waiting: standing in line, dentists, haircuts Arousing activities: sex, scary movies, exercise
Social anxiety and shyness	*Situations that trigger fear of humiliation or embarrassment* Interpersonal contact with others: conversations, dating, meeting new people, parties, interviews, meetings, being assertive Being the center of attention: public speaking, performing, playing sports, writing in public, eating or drinking in front of others
Generalized anxiety and worry	*Situations that trigger particular worries* Worries about money: opening bills, spending money Worries about work: being behind on e-mails, having a meeting with the boss, a fast-approaching deadline Worries about family: child doing poorly on a test, spouse arriving home from work, child has a cold Worries about health: going to the doctor, reading about medical illnesses, seeing a TV show on a particular health problem, experiencing pain, eating unhealthy foods Worries about being on time: bad traffic, leaving home without enough time to spare Worries about not sleeping: lying in bed, drinking coffee
Obsessive–compulsive concerns	*Situations that trigger obsessional thoughts, urges, and images* Contamination concerns: touching "contaminated" objects such as money, doorknobs, other people, elevator buttons, and other items; coming into contact with "toxins," including detergents, chemicals, gasoline, and other such products

table 2.1 *(cont.)*

Anxiety problem	Common situational triggers
Obsessive–compulsive concerns *(cont.)*	Irrational concerns about acting aggressively: being around certain people (for example, children) if worried about acting aggressively toward them, being around objects that could be used to hurt others (for example, knives)
	Fears of particular words or images: hearing feared words, seeing feared images, talking about topics that are related to feared words or images
	Concerns about making mistakes: writing letters, taking tests, having conversations, or engaging in other activities in which feared mistakes may occur
Anxiety related to a history of trauma	*Situations that trigger a fear of particular types of trauma recurring, either in reality or in memory* Sexual assault: being around men, being alone, being sexually intimate, going out at night, watching movies with violent scenes, visiting the place where the assault took place, talking about the assault
	Car accident: driving, being a passenger in a car, allowing loved ones to drive or be in a car, talking about the accident, walking on the road where the accident occurred, watching movies depicting people driving fast
	Combat-related trauma: being in public places, talking about the trauma, being around other war veterans, hearing loud noises such as thunder or fireworks, seeing guns
Specific phobias: animals	*Situations where feared animals are often encountered* Dogs: seeing dogs, being close to a dog, visiting people who have dogs, touching dogs, walking in parks or around the neighborhood, visiting pet stores
	Snakes: seeing snakes at the zoo, in a pet store, or in the wild; being in areas where there may be a snake; seeing snakes in photos or on television; talking about snakes
	Spiders and bugs: going outside; gardening; going into basements; seeing spiders and bugs live, on film, or in photos
Specific phobias: blood and needles	*Situations where blood and needles may be encountered* Blood: seeing surgery, having surgery, watching childbirth, watching medical TV shows and movies, being in a hospital or doctor's office
	Needles: giving blood, having a blood test, having an injection, watching a blood test or an injection, going to the dentist

(cont.)

table 2.1 (cont.)

Anxiety problem	Common situational triggers
Specific phobias: other situations	*Situations where other fear triggers may be encountered* Enclosed places: tunnels, small rooms, small cars, airplanes, hugging, blankets covering the head, shower stalls, basements, closets, crawl spaces, garages, windowless rooms, crowded spaces
	Flying: being on airplanes
	Driving: driving on highways, driving on city streets, making left-hand turns, parking, driving in high places
	Heights: ladders, rooftops, tall buildings, glass elevators, looking down over a railing, balconies, stadiums, bridges, amusement park rides
	Storms: thunder, lightning, rain, snow
	Water: swimming in pools, lakes, or the ocean, taking baths
	Vomiting: eating certain foods, not knowing where a bathroom is, being around young children, being around sick people, reading in a car, being on a boat
	Choking: eating certain foods, swallowing pills
	Tests and exams: taking tests, studying for tests, taking courses that include tests, enrolling in college

each problem separately (Form 2.1 includes space for three different anxiety problems; use extra paper if you need more space). If you can't find your anxiety problem in the table, just write it in on the form.

What Variables Affect Your Fear?

Now that you have categorized the situations that trigger your anxiety and fear, you need to learn to recognize the specific circumstances that affect your level of fear and anxiety in these situations. If you fear driving, for example, your level of fear may depend on all sorts of factors, including the type of car you're driving, whether it's daytime or nighttime, how tired you are, and how slippery the roads are. Why is this so important to know? In Chapters 5 and 6, you'll learn about a powerful strategy to reduce fear by exposing yourself to the situations you fear; you can influence how much fear you experience during exposure therapy by changing the variables that affect your fear in the situations in which you practice your exposures.

Table 2.2 includes some examples of variables that influence fear and anxiety for various types of anxiety problems. Look over the table, then generate a list of the

form 2.1	**Situational Triggers for My Anxiety Problems**
Anxiety problem	**Situational triggers**
1.	
2.	
3.	

table 2.2. **Variables That Often Affect Fear and Anxiety Levels for Various Anxiety Problems**

Anxiety problem	Examples of variables that may affect fear and anxiety
Panic disorder and agoraphobia	Driving: right lane versus left lane, window open versus closed, alone versus accompanied, amount of traffic, distance between highway exits
	Buses and trains: distance between your seat and the door, distance between stops
	Crowded places: how crowded, how far you are from the door, alone versus accompanied
	Enclosed places: size of space, presence of windows
Social anxiety and shyness	Aspects of the other person or people: age, sex, how familiar you are with them, whether they are attractive, smart, confident, successful, aggressive
	Aspects of the situation: lighting, how formal the situation is, number of people present, position (for example, standing, sitting, or whatever), whether you have been drinking, how long you're stuck in the situation, the specific activity (for example, eating messy foods versus sitting quietly)
Generalized anxiety and worry	How you feel physically (for example, fatigue)
	Whether you can get reassurance or check to make sure your worries are not true
Obsessive–compulsive concerns	Whether you can use some sort of compulsion or safety behavior to decrease your anxiety (for example, checking, counting, cleaning, washing)
	Whether you can get reassurance from someone else
Anxiety related to a history of trauma	Sexual assault: whether you're alone when leaving the house, how familiar you are with the man you're spending time with, whether it's dark or light out when going to the mall
	Car accident: speed of traffic, size of your car, type of road (for example, highway versus city street), amount of traffic, weather, dark versus light
Specific phobias: animals	Size of the animal, way in which the animal moves (fast versus slow, jerky versus smooth movements), whether the animal is restrained (for example, dog on a leash, spider in a jar), color of the animal, whether the animal looks "mean" or angry
Specific phobias: blood and needles	Blood: format of the presentation of blood (for example, in a bag, in a tube, on a person, on TV)

table 2.2 *(cont.)*

Anxiety problem	Examples of variables that may affect fear and anxiety
Specific phobias: blood and needles *(cont.)*	Needles: size of the needle, location of the needle site (for example, blood test in middle of arm, injection in top of arm, finger prick blood test, dentist's needle in the mouth), environment of the exposure (for example, hospital versus home)
Specific phobias: other situations	Enclosed places: size of space, presence of windows, temperature, stuffiness
	Flying: size of plane, duration of flight, airline, weather, amount of turbulence, whether other passengers seem "dangerous"
	Driving: type of road, whether the radio is on, night versus day, amount of traffic, speed of traffic, whether someone is following you too closely, whether you're tired, whether you're alone
	Heights: distance from the ground, open height versus closed in (for example, balcony versus window), distance from the edge, amount of movement around you (for example, other people walking around)
	Storms: severity of the storm
	Water: depth of the water, natural versus man-made (for example, lake versus swimming pool)
	Vomiting: type of food being eaten, amount of motion on the boat or car trip
	Choking: size of the object to be swallowed (for example, large pill versus small pill), type of food being eaten (for example, steak versus pudding)
	Tests and exams: familiarity of the material, amount of studying, format of the test (for example, essay versus multiple choice)

variables that influence your fear and record them on Form 2.2. Again, you may include examples from the table, but try to come up with other examples as well. If you have more than one anxiety problem, list relevant variables for each problem (Form 2.2 includes space for three different anxiety problems, but use extra paper if that isn't enough). If your anxiety problem isn't included in the table, list it on the form with its situational triggers.

What Do You Feel When You Are Anxious or Frightened?

In all likelihood, your fear and anxiety are associated with a range of physical symptoms and sensations. When we feel anxious or frightened, we become physically aroused. The arousal may take the form of a racing or pounding heart, sweating, trembling or

form 2.2	Variables That Affect My Fear and Anxiety
Anxiety problem	**Variables that affect my fear and anxiety**
1.	
2.	
3.	

shaking, shortness of breath, choking feelings, tightness or discomfort in the chest, nausea or butterflies in the stomach, dizziness, unsteadiness, faintness, feelings of unreality, feeling detached as if outside your body, numbness or tingling sensations, hot flushes, chills, muscle tension or tightness, aches and pains, visual distortions (for example, blurred vision), as well as other uncomfortable feelings.

Is it important to be aware of the sensations you experience when feeling anxious? The answer to that question depends on how concerned you are about them. If you're not concerned at all about the physical sensations of arousal, it may not be important to spend much time trying to figure out which sensations you experience. On the other hand, if you're frightened by the sensations or if you do find them bothersome, knowing which sensations you experience will be important when you begin to use specific strategies described in later chapters to combat your reactions. If the physical symptoms of arousal frighten you, it is important to learn different ways of responding to them.

It will also be helpful for you to recognize whether you experience panic attacks in the context of the situations you fear. Fainting is common among people who have phobias of blood or needles, for instance, but very uncommon for people with other types of anxiety problems. Panic attacks are common among most people with anxiety-based problems.

Form 2.3 provides space for you to record the physical sensations you experience when feeling anxious or frightened. Think about how these sensations might vary depending on the type of anxiety problem you're experiencing. You may feel your heart race when speaking in front of groups, for example, and muscle tension and headaches when worrying about your finances. This form provides space for you to record your typical physical sensations for up to three different anxiety problems. Again, use extra paper if you need it.

What Are Your Anxiety-Provoking Thoughts?

Your fear and anxiety are greatly influenced by the sorts of beliefs, thoughts, assumptions, and predictions that you hold about the situations, sensations, thoughts, and images that trigger your anxiety. Chances are that when you're feeling anxious or frightened, you're predicting that something negative will occur or that the situations you fear are dangerous in some way. Are you aware of your anxious thoughts? Often people have a hard time describing their thoughts and predictions because they're so quick and automatic, almost like a habit. Do your best in this early stage in your treatment to identify the anxious thoughts that influence your fear. In Chapter 4 you'll have an opportunity to revisit this issue in detail.

Table 2.3 provides examples of typical anxious thoughts that are associated with a wide range of common anxiety-based problems. Note that some of these anxious predictions have to do with the external object or situation (for example, "The dog will bite me"), whereas others reflect concern about our own beliefs (for example, "If I think about hurting my child, that means I'm likely to do it") or our own physical sensations (for example, "If my heart races too quickly, I'll drop dead of a heart attack").

form 2.3	**Physical Sensations Associated with My Fear and Anxiety**
Anxiety problem	**Physical sensations**
1.	History of panic attacks? (sudden onset of fear, with four or more symptoms; see Chapter 1) Yes☐ No☐ History of fainting? Yes☐ No☐
2.	History of panic attacks? (sudden onset of fear, with four or more symptoms; see Chapter 1) Yes☐ No☐ History of fainting? Yes☐ No☐
3.	History of panic attacks? (sudden onset of fear, with four or more symptoms; see Chapter 1) Yes☐ No☐ History of fainting? Yes☐ No☐

table 2.3. **Common Anxious Thoughts Associated with Various Anxiety Problems**

Anxiety problem	Examples of common anxiety-provoking thoughts
Panic disorder and agoraphobia	"I won't be able to cope if I have a panic attack in the theater." "I'm guaranteed to panic if I go for a drive." "My panic attack may never end." "I will lose control or go crazy during a panic attack." "If my heart races too quickly, I will drop dead of a heart attack." "I will faint during a panic attack." "I will vomit or lose bowel control during a panic attack." "Panic and anxiety are signs of weakness." "People will think I'm weak or strange if they find out about my anxiety."
Social anxiety and shyness	"People will think there is something wrong with me if they notice my shaking, blushing, or sweating." "It would be terrible to make a mistake in front of other people." "It's important for everybody to like me." "I will make a fool of myself during the presentation." "People are very critical and judgmental." "I am incompetent."
Generalized anxiety and worry	"I will run out of money and won't be able to care for myself." "My children will get into trouble if I don't take steps to protect them." "If my family members show even mild physical symptoms, it could be a sign of serious illness." "I won't be able to cope with the stress of work or school." "If I don't get enough sleep, I won't be able to function the next day." "Worrying may drive me crazy." "Worrying helps me prevent bad things from happening."
Obsessive–compulsive concerns	"Touching 'contaminated' objects will make me sick." "If I think about hurting my child, that means I'm likely to do it." "If I have a violent thought, that means I'm a bad person."

(cont.)

table 2.3 *(cont.)*

Anxiety problem	Examples of common anxiety-provoking thoughts
Obsessive–compulsive concerns *(cont.)*	"If I have an inappropriate sexual thought, that means I'm likely to act on it."
	"If I make even a small mistake, terrible things will happen."
	"I can't throw anything away in case I need it later."
	"If things are out of order, I will be so overwhelmed with fear and anxiety that I will not be able to function."
Anxiety related to a history of trauma	"If I don't take steps to protect myself, I will experience another trauma."
	"I should have been able to prevent my trauma from happening in the first place."
	"The world is a dangerous place."
	"If I allow myself to think about my trauma, I may lose control or go completely crazy."
Specific phobias: animals	"The dog will bite me."
	"I will drop dead from fear if I see a snake."
	"The bird will sense my fear and fly toward me."
	"The spider will crawl on me."
Specific phobias: blood and needles	"The needle will be painful."
	"I will faint if I see blood."
	"I will get AIDS from a blood test."
	"I won't be able to cope if I need surgery."
Specific phobias: other situations	"I won't be able to escape from an enclosed place."
	"I will run out of air and suffocate on an elevator."
	"The airplane will crash or get hijacked."
	"My car will crash."
	"If I stand on the high balcony, it will collapse."
	"If I get dizzy in a high place, I'll fall."
	"In a high place, I will become overwhelmed with an urge to jump."
	"I will be struck by lightning during a storm."
	"I will drown if I go into the water."

table 2.3 *(cont.)*

Anxiety problem	Examples of common anxiety-provoking thoughts
Specific phobias: other situations *(cont.)*	"If I vomit, the experience will be so unpleasant that I won't be able to cope." "I will choke and die if I eat meat." "I will do poorly on my exam and fail my course."

Once you have reviewed the examples in the table, complete Form 2.4 by recording the anxiety-provoking thoughts and predictions that run through your head when you're feeling anxious or frightened. The best way to identify your anxious thoughts is to ask yourself questions like "What am I afraid will happen?" and "What would be so terrible about being in the situation I fear?" The form provides space to record your anxious thoughts for three different anxiety problems. If you need more space, feel free to use extra paper.

What Situations and Objects Do You Avoid?

The urge to avoid feared situations can be very strong, maybe even overwhelming. Naturally, if you're convinced that a situation is dangerous or threatening, you'll do what you can to avoid it. What situations and objects do you avoid? In all likelihood, the list of situations that you avoid will be very similar to the list of situations and objects that trigger your fear, which you recorded on Form 2.1. Having a comprehensive list of situations you avoid will be useful when you begin to plan exposure practices in Chapters 5 and 6.

Form 2.5 can be used to record the situations you tend to avoid because of your anxiety and fear, as well as how frequently you avoid each situation. As with the other forms in this chapter, this one provides space to record information for up to three different anxiety problems and you should add more if you need to. For each anxiety problem, list the situations and objects you tend to avoid in the second column (referring back to your list of anxiety triggers on Form 2.1 will be helpful). In the third column, record a number from 0 to 100 to represent how frequently you avoid each situation (0 means that you never avoid the situation; 50 means that you avoid the situation about half the time; and 100 means that you avoid the situation completely).

How Do You Protect Yourself from Danger in the Situations You Fear?

Sometimes it's impossible to avoid a situation completely, and yet the urge to self-protect is very strong. Therefore, when people are exposed to situations they fear, they often rely on safety behaviors to protect themselves. In the case of obsessive–compulsive disorder

form 2.4	**Anxiety-Provoking Thoughts Associated with My Anxiety Problems**
Anxiety problem	**Anxiety-provoking thoughts**
1.	
2.	
3.	

form 2.5	Situations I Avoid	
Anxiety problem	**Situations and objects I avoid**	**Frequency of avoidance (0–100)**
1.		
2.		
3.		

(OCD), compulsions such as checking, washing, cleaning, counting, and repeating are actually safety behaviors that people with OCD use to try to guard against their fears. All the anxiety disorders are associated with safety behaviors to varying degrees. Table 2.4 includes examples of safety behaviors for a wide range of common anxiety problems.

After looking over the examples in the table, generate a list of your own safety behaviors and record them in Form 2.6. You guessed it: you may include examples from the table, but please try to come up with other examples too. If you have more than one anxiety problem, list your triggers for each problem in Form 2.6, using extra paper if needed.

What Internal Experiences Do You Fear and Avoid?

As described earlier, for most people, anxiety problems are triggered by particular situations, such as driving, public speaking, being in high places, or confronting a feared animal. But people are also often anxious about their own private experiences, including the physical sensations they experience and the thoughts, images, urges, and memories that run through their minds.

Fear of Physical Sensations

Fear of physical sensations is very common among people with certain types of anxiety disorders. For example:

+ A person with panic disorder may be fearful of sensations that may be mistaken for a heart attack (racing heart, breathlessness, sweating), being about to faint (dizziness, lightheadedness), or being about to go "crazy" or lose control (feelings of unreality, feeling detached from oneself).
+ A person with social anxiety may be fearful of blushing, shaking, sweating, or showing other visible signs of anxiety in front of other people.
+ A person with a fear of heights may be fearful of getting dizzy because it might lead to falling.
+ A person who fears driving may be anxious about feeling lightheaded because it might lead to a car accident.
+ A person with claustrophobia may fear that sensations of breathlessness in an enclosed place are an indication of suffocation.

In the first column of Form 2.7 is a list of physical sensations that often occur when people feel anxious or frightened, as well as for other reasons. In the second column, record how frightened you would be to experience the sensation in general (in a situation that's normally calm for you—for example, feeling dizzy while watching TV). Use any number ranging from 0 to 100, where 0 equals no fear at all and 100 equals as frightened as you can imagine being. In the third column, record a number to indicate

table 2.4. **Common Safety Behaviors Used with Various Anxiety Problems**

Anxiety problem	Examples of common safety behaviors
Panic disorder and agoraphobia	Sitting in the aisle seat in a theater to facilitate a quick escape
	Always having a "safe person" around when going into feared situations
	Carrying medication in case a panic attack comes on
	Frequently checking your pulse to make sure your heart isn't beating too quickly
	Sitting down and resting when panic feelings begin
	Cleaning the house as a distraction from panic sensations
Social anxiety and shyness	Wearing makeup to hide blushing
	Wearing light clothing to hide sweating in public
	Eating in dimly lit restaurants so people won't notice you blushing
	Overpreparing for presentations
	Avoiding certain topics of conversation
	Avoiding eye contact when talking to others
Generalized anxiety and worry	Leaving home extra early for appointments so there's no chance of being late
	Phoning your children frequently to make sure they're okay
	Not carrying money or wearing jewelry for fear of being mugged, even in areas that most people would consider safe
	Not buying things you can easily afford for fear of one day having no money
	Exercising excessively to prevent possible health problems
Obsessive–compulsive concerns	Wearing gloves when touching things that may be "contaminated"
	Excessive hand washing to clean off possible contamination
	Repeated checking to make sure that work was done correctly
	Engaging in superstitious behaviors to prevent bad things from happening
	Making sure things are organized perfectly to avoid feeling a sense of discomfort or incompleteness
	Repeating positive words or phrases to yourself to replace frightening thoughts that pop into your mind

(cont.)

table 2.4 *(cont.)*

Anxiety problem	Examples of common safety behaviors
Anxiety related to a history of trauma	Carrying pepper spray to protect yourself from possible assault
	Driving extra slowly to avoid a possible car accident
	Walking with your back to the wall in public places to prevent the possibility of being attacked from behind
Specific phobias: animals	Checking for dogs through the window before leaving the house to go for a walk
	Carrying an umbrella or a stick to protect yourself from harmless snakes while out walking
	Making sure that the basement is brightly lit before going downstairs in order to see any spiders or insects that might be there
Specific phobias: blood and needles	Lying down during a blood test to avoid becoming faint
	Looking away during an injection
Specific phobias: other situations	Asking the doctor to leave the examination room door open during a medical exam to avoid feeling closed in
	Flying in business class to avoid feeling closed in
	Driving only in the right lane to make it easy to pull over if necessary
	Driving in the left lane on bridges to protect yourself from seeing over the edge
	Staying in the basement with the lights on and the music turned up to avoid seeing lightning and hearing thunder during a storm
	Overpreparing for tests and exams

how frightened you would be to experience the sensation in a situation that normally makes you feel anxious (for example, feeling dizzy in a high place). In later chapters, you'll learn some strategies to overcome any fear you experience in response to physical sensations.

Fear of Thoughts, Images, Urges, and Memories

Sometimes people fear their own thoughts. In other words, they respond to their own thoughts, memories, urges, and images as if they are dangerous. They may do everything

My Safety Behaviors

Anxiety problem	Safety behaviors
1.	
2.	
3.	

they can to prevent themselves from having these thoughts, which just makes the problem worse. Examples of people who fear their thoughts include:

+ A man with obsessive–compulsive disorder who worries that if he thinks about hurting a loved one, he's likely to do it
+ A woman who fears that having a negative thought about God pop into her head means that she's a bad person
+ A person who fears that if she thinks about her worries too much, she won't be able to sleep
+ A person with a driving phobia who fears that having impulses to drive off a bridge means he will act on these urges
+ A person who was sexually assaulted who is afraid to allow herself to remember the rape because she might not be able to cope with the memories

form 2.7 — **Fear of Physical Sensations**		
Sensation	**Fear of sensation in general (0–100)**	**Fear of sensation when in a feared situation (0–100)**
Racing or pounding heart		
Chest tightness or pain		
Dizziness, faintness, lightheadedness		
Breathlessness or smothering sensations		
Sweating		
Hot flushes or chills		
Numbness or tingling sensations		
Nausea or abdominal discomfort		
Choking feelings or a tightness in the throat		
Blurred vision		
Feeling unreal or detached		

On the blank lines, describe any thoughts you tend to experience that you find frightening because it feels as though the thoughts themselves might be dangerous or threatening. You may also record any memories that frighten you, as well as any scary images, impulses, or urges. (If you're not afraid of these thoughts, if you make no effort to suppress them, and you don't believe that your thoughts, images, or impulses are dangerous, you may skip this exercise.)

_____

_____

_____

_____

_____

_____

_____

Are You Experiencing Any Other Difficulties?

Now we'd like you to reflect on whether there are any other difficulties in your life that may affect your ability to work on your anxiety problem, such as other emotional problems (for example, depression), substance use problems (for example, alcohol or drug abuse), medical illnesses (for example, heart disease, chronic pain), interpersonal problems (for example, relationship difficulties), and life stresses (for example, hectic work schedule, significant financial problems). Having other problems doesn't mean you shouldn't try to overcome your anxiety at this time. If the other problems are so severe or impairing that you can't imagine focusing on your anxiety right now, however, you should work on the other issues first and then come back to the anxiety.

In the space below, record any other difficulties that might have an effect on your ability to follow the program described in this book. Describe whether you can work around these difficulties or put them off to the side in order to work on your anxiety.

_____

_____

_____

_____

_____

_____

The Importance of Ongoing Assessment

The process of self-assessment is important for developing a treatment plan up front, and it's also useful for assessing whether treatment is working down the road. You should refer back to your responses on the forms in this chapter from time to time to see how things have changed. As you work through the strategies in this book, you will find it helpful to know if your anxiety is still triggered by the same sorts of situations, feelings, and thoughts that triggered your anxiety at the start of your treatment. You'll also want to know whether your anxiety-related sensations, thoughts, and behaviors have changed over time, and whether your anxiety interferes with your life in the same ways it did when you began to work through this book.

If you were on a plan to lose weight, chances are you might weigh yourself from time to time to keep a record of your progress. In the same way, it will be helpful to keep track of your progress in this program by completing Form 2.8. Each week (ideally on the same day), complete the three ratings across one row of this form. If you're working on more than one anxiety problem, complete a separate copy of this form for each problem.

Conclusion

In this chapter, you explored all facets of your anxiety problem as a first step toward planning your treatment. Specifically, you identified the situations, objects, sensations, and thoughts that trigger your anxiety, as well as the ways in which you respond to your anxiety-provoking triggers. You also began to monitor the severity of your anxiety problem, a process that you will continue through the treatment process. The information you gathered in this chapter will be used as you prepare to overcome your anxiety problems in the remaining chapters in this book. Good luck!

Weekly Record of Anxiety

Problem _____

Date	Average overall anxiety in the past week (1–100; 0 = no anxiety, 100 = very severe anxiety)	Overall severity of the specified problem (0–100; 0 = no problem at all, and 100 = very severe)	Overall change since the beginning (-10 to +10; -10 = much worse, 0 = no change, +10 = much better)

3

Getting Ready for Treatment

Working through this book will give you the tools you need to confront and overcome the anxiety that has been holding you back. But it will demand something of you: it will take your full attention, your desire and willingness to change, and a considerable amount of your time. This chapter will help you to decide whether you're committed to making these changes today and to get ready to take the steps to overcome your anxiety. As you work through this chapter, you'll be setting goals. If you suffer from several different anxiety problems, you'll need to decide which problems you want to work on first and which can wait. You'll also explore the options of working through this program on your own, with the help of a close friend or family member, or with a professional therapist. Finally, strategies for choosing among various treatment approaches and for developing a comprehensive treatment plan will be discussed.

Is Now the Best Time to Start This Program?

You might feel a bit nervous about going forward with this program and worry about how you'll find the time to practice the exercises recommended in this book. That's perfectly normal. But if you feel you can't make these commitments, we advise you not to undertake the program now, as it may mean compromising the outcome of your treatment or feeling disappointed or discouraged by your results. If you're ready for it, there is every reason to believe that you will experience significant improvements in your anxiety, just as most people who used the strategies described in this book have.

Here are some issues to consider in deciding whether this is the best time for you to start this program: (1) the severity of your problem, (2) the potential costs and benefits to you of overcoming your problem, and (3) potential obstacles and challenges to overcoming your problem.

How Much of a Problem Is Your Anxiety?

Daniel is terrified of driving, especially on highways. Because of his fear, he can't take the sorts of trips that he and his girlfriend would love to take, and he has turned down several jobs that would have required him to drive to work. He relies on public transit and on help from his friends and family to get around. Daniel is embarrassed by his fear, and he wishes he could be more at ease when driving.

Nisha is very nervous when speaking in front of groups, so she avoids public speaking at all costs. She works in customer service, so public speaking never comes up in her job. She only encounters the possibility of public speaking every few years when she is asked to make a toast or give a short speech at a party or wedding (which she always turns down). Nisha rarely thinks about her fear of public speaking, and it doesn't really bother her.

Clearly, Daniel is a better candidate for treatment than Nisha. Daniel's anxiety is causing a lot of problems in his personal and professional life, which means he's likely to be motivated to get help and to work hard to overcome his fear. For Nisha, however, treatment may be a lot of work without much payoff in terms of improving her quality of life. Getting treatment is unlikely to be a priority for Nisha at this time.

It's perfectly normal to feel anxious from time to time, to fear certain objects and situations, and to avoid places and situations that trigger your fear. Anxiety and fear only become a problem when they're bothersome to you or stop you from doing things that are important to you. To consider whether your anxiety and fears are a problem, answer the following questions:

1. How often do significant anxiety and fear come up in your day-to-day life?

   _____

   _____

2. How much does it bother you that you have difficulties with anxiety and fear?

   _____

   _____

3. In what ways do your anxiety, fear, avoidance, and safety behaviors interfere with your life, including work, school, relationships with family and friends, intimate relationships, health, hobbies and leisure activities, management of your finances, management of household responsibilities, religious expression, or other areas?

   _____

   _____

   _____

   _____

If your anxiety comes up frequently, is bothersome to you, and interferes with your life, it's time to do something about it! And you probably wouldn't have picked up this book if you didn't already know that.

What Are the Costs and Benefits of Overcoming Your Anxiety?

If overcoming your anxiety is associated with many costs and relatively few benefits, you may decide not to work on the problem right now. On the other hand, if the benefits of overcoming your anxiety outweigh the costs, then tackling the problem now may be a good idea. Table 3.1 includes examples of possible costs and benefits of going through this treatment. Form 3.1 provides you with space to record your own list of costs and benefits.

What Are the Obstacles and Challenges That May Get in the Way?

Take this opportunity to identify any obstacles that may interfere with your treatment, and think about possible solutions. We'll discuss some common challenges, as well as ideas for overcoming them. At the end of this section, you'll have an opportunity to identify obstacles that may negatively affect your own treatment and to brainstorm possible solutions (see Form 3.2).

Not Enough Time to Devote to the Problem

One of the most common reasons why people put off treatment is a lack of time. To get the most out of this treatment, you need to spend some time working on the problem almost every day—whether it's reading this book, completing various forms and worksheets, and/or using the strategies described in the book. The amount of time you need will depend on the types of problems you're working on, the number of different anxiety issues you have, the severity of your anxiety and related issues, and how quickly you respond to the treatment. Some people are able to overcome their anxiety with relatively little effort (maybe with just a few hours of a certain practice), but most people will need a few weeks or months of hard work (such as practicing for an hour or two almost every day).

Even if you feel there are too many demands on your time, you may be able to adapt the treatment to suit your schedule. Many of the strategies can be used at various levels of intensity, depending on the time you have available. For example, if you're using exposure-based strategies to overcome a fear of driving, you can practice driving several evenings per week for an hour or so, and chances are you will notice that you're feeling less fearful after several weeks or months. Alternatively, you can take a couple of weeks off work and make driving practice your full-time job. By practicing driving all day long for a week or two, you might notice just as much improvement as the person in the previous scenario.

You will see that many of the strategies described in this book can be integrated

table 3.1. **Examples of Possible Costs and Benefits of Overcoming Your Anxiety**

Possible costs of treating your anxiety	Possible benefits of treating your anxiety
Aspects of the therapy may be time-consuming (for example, exposure practices and completion of monitoring forms).	You may be able to enter situations that you currently avoid.
Aspects of the therapy may be boring or tedious (for example, completing forms and diaries, concentrating as you read this book).	You may be able to do things that are important to you so you can live a life that is more consistent with your personal values.
Aspects of the therapy may be frightening (for example, confronting feared situations).	You may feel calmer, more relaxed, and happier.
The therapy may cost money, particularly if you decide to see a therapist.	Your self-esteem may improve.
The therapy may have an impact on your friends' and family members' time (for example, if you need them to help with certain aspects of the treatment).	You may be less frightened of the objects, situations, sensations, thoughts, or images that currently make you anxious.
Overcoming your anxiety may lead to a reduction in attention, support, concern, or help from others (especially your family).	You may spend less time on safety behaviors, compulsions, and efforts to avoid feeling uncomfortable.
Getting over your anxiety may mean that you'll have to start doing things that you don't want to do (for example, if anxiety has prevented you from doing certain tasks that you don't enjoy, such as working, shopping, running errands, doing housework).	You may no longer feel embarrassed about your problem or have to hide it from others.
	You may be able to perform more effectively at work or school.
	The quality of your relationships and friendships may improve.
	You may be able to pursue new relationships, jobs, and other activities from which your anxiety previously held you back.
	You may have an opportunity to focus on things that are important to you other than your anxiety, but that you didn't have the chance to focus on before.

form 3.1 **Costs and Benefits of Overcoming My Anxiety**

Thinking about your own anxiety and your own life, record the costs and benefits of working through this program to overcome your particular anxiety problems.

Costs of overcoming my anxiety	Benefits of overcoming my anxiety
• _____	• _____
_____	_____
_____	_____
• _____	• _____
_____	_____
_____	_____
• _____	• _____
_____	_____
_____	_____
• _____	• _____
_____	_____
_____	_____
• _____	• _____
_____	_____
_____	_____
• _____	• _____
_____	_____
_____	_____
• _____	• _____
_____	_____
_____	_____
• _____	• _____
_____	_____
_____	_____

form 3.2	**Obstacles and Challenges to My Treatment**

In the first column, record any obstacles or challenges that you anticipate may affect your treatment as you work through this program. In the second column, record possible ways in which you can overcome each obstacle.

Obstacle or challenge	Solution

From *The Anti-Anxiety Workbook* by Martin M. Antony and Peter J. Norton. Copyright 2009 by The Guilford Press.

into your regular routine so they don't take up extra time. Schedule your homework practices just as you would any other activities or appointments in your life. If they're written into your schedule, you will be more likely to find the time to get them done.

Serious Stresses in Your Life

If you are currently experiencing significant ongoing stress, it may be particularly difficult for you to devote the energy needed to overcoming your anxiety problems right now. The kind of stresses that may pose a problem include extreme work stress, such as too much work, tight deadlines, a difficult boss, the threat of losing your job, or unemployment; relationship problems like frequent arguments, a recent breakup, or an abusive relationship; family stress, such as illness, death, legal problems, or child-care issues; and other stresses such as financial hardship, upcoming exams, moving, or medical problems.

If the stress you're experiencing is short term, consider waiting to begin this treatment until after it has passed. But if it's chronic and likely to continue for a while, you may as well begin working on your anxiety now, particularly if you think you can focus on the problem despite the stress. The good news is that some of the strategies discussed in this book (particularly those in Chapters 4, 9, 10, and 11) have the bonus of helping you manage the stress in your life more effectively, in addition to helping with your anxiety problems.

Financial Challenges

Some of the treatment strategies discussed in this book may cost money. It may be difficult to overcome a fear of flying, for example, without practicing flying on airplanes. Similarly, overcoming a fear of eating in public restaurants requires you to practice dining in public. If you decide to use this book in the context of therapy with a mental health professional, you'll also need to consider the therapist's fees (depending on your insurance coverage). If your finances are tight, you may need to limit how much you practice the exercises that aren't free or inexpensive.

Lack of Support from Friends or Family

A lack of support from friends or family members can make it more difficult to overcome problems with anxiety (or any problem, for that matter). If friends and family trivialize your problems, tease you for feeling anxious, or become angry because you aren't able to do things that frighten you, these behaviors can undermine your motivation. Some of the practices described in this book work best if done with the help of a friend or family member, which will be impossible if you don't feel you can approach one for help. If this is the case, you should be reassured to know that many people are able to overcome their anxiety problems without such outside support.

If you're fortunate enough to have the help of friends or family, though, take advantage of it as you carry out the treatment. Have your close friends or family members who will be involved read Chapter 14, which provides suggestions for how they can help with the treatment process. They may also find it helpful to read other sections of this book.

Setting Goals

An important strategy for keeping your treatment on track is to set goals. Setting goals will help you select appropriate treatment methods and make it easier to determine whether treatment is working (that is, whether your goals are being met). Reminding yourself of your goals on a regular basis also keeps your motivation strong as you work to reduce your anxiety. At the end of this section, you will have an opportunity to record your goals for treatment (see Form 3.3).

Specific versus Broad Goals

Although it's okay to have a few broader goals, most of your goals should be as specific as possible. This makes it easier for you to select particular treatment strategies to meet your goals and to assess whether you're getting closer to meeting them. Here are some examples to help you understand the difference between specific and broad goals.

Examples of Specific Goals

+ To stop having unexpected panic attacks
+ To sit in the same room as a dog without feeling anxious
+ To make at least three new friends over the next year
+ To apply for at least 10 new jobs over the next month
+ To leave the house each day regardless of how anxious I am feeling
+ To stop all compulsive washing
+ To cut down the frequency of worrying about my children by at least 50%
+ To sleep at least 7 hours through the night
+ To drive from work to home with minimal anxiety

Examples of Broad Goals

+ To be less anxious and worried
+ To be more satisfied with my job
+ To reduce the frequency of anxiety-provoking thoughts
+ To be happy
+ To feel calm
+ To have better relationships

Short-Term versus Long-Term Goals

As you develop your list of goals, include examples for the short term, the medium term, and the long term. Short-term goals might include objectives that you would like to accomplish in the first month of your treatment; medium-term goals might include those targeted for the next few months; and longer term goals might include those that you intend to fulfill over the next few years. Of course, you can develop goals that cover any time period you want, from a few minutes from now to the next 30 years. Below are some examples of short-term, medium-term, and long-term goals for Leigh, who suffers from OCD (specifically, she feels the need to check her work repeatedly), as well as anxiety in social situations, occasional unexpected panic attacks, and occasional bouts of moderate depression.

Leigh's Short-Term Goals (for the Next 4 Weeks)

✦ To reduce her compulsive checking (for example, locks, stoves) to less than 1 hour per day
✦ To spend at least 2 hours per day working on her anxiety problems
✦ To begin thinking less anxiously when in social situations

Leigh's Medium-Term Goals (for the Next 4 Months)

✦ To eliminate all compulsive checking
✦ To be able to leave home without experiencing an intense urge to check the locks and stoves more than once
✦ To no longer experience panic attacks
✦ To feel less anxious in social situations such as parties, work meetings, meeting new people, and dating
✦ To look for a new job (to apply for at least five jobs per week until finding one)

Leigh's Long-Term Goals (for 2 Years from Now)

✦ To be in a long-term relationship
✦ To have a new job that she enjoys
✦ To maintain the gains she has made with respect to her social anxiety, OCD, and panic attacks
✦ To no longer feel depressed

Multiple Anxiety Problems: Deciding Where to Start

Based on the description of various anxiety problems in Chapter 1, the information you gathered in Chapter 2, and the goals you set in this chapter, you should have a good idea of the types of anxiety problems you are currently experiencing. Before going any further, take a few minutes to record up to eight different problems you have with anxiety. These can include situations you fear, problems with obsessions or compulsions, tendencies to worry excessively, or any other anxiety problems.

Next, rank these in terms of *importance,* with 1 being the problem you want to work on first. Your rankings can be based on how severe the problem is, how much you want to overcome it, or any other factors that make it important for you to overcome it. Most people choose to work first on the problems that are most distressing and that interfere the most in their lives. This information can be recorded on Form 3.4, which includes a sample of a completed form, as well as one with space for you to record your responses.

Including a Helper or "Co-Therapist"

Although it's certainly not necessary to include a family member or close friend as a helper or "co-therapist," doing so may be helpful for a number of reasons. First, your

form 3.3	**Treatment Goals**
	Record your goals for treatment. Be as specific as possible.

Period	Goals
Short-term (next 4 weeks)	• _____ _____ • _____ _____ • _____ _____ • _____ _____
Medium-term (next 4 months)	• _____ _____ • _____ _____ • _____ _____ • _____ _____
Long-term (next 2 years)	• _____ _____ • _____ _____ • _____ _____ • _____ _____

Anxiety Problem List

Sample Completed Form

Anxiety problem	Ranking
I am very anxious in social situations, including parties, meeting new people, and being the center of attention.	1
I feel panicky whenever I think about a traumatic car accident that I experienced almost 7 years ago. I avoid driving and any situations that remind me of the accident—even talking about it makes me feel that I may lose control.	2
I am afraid of flying, though I almost never need to fly and I don't care too much about this fear.	4
I tend to worry too much about almost everything, including work, my children, finances, and my husband. I worry even when everything is okay.	3

Your Anxiety Problem List

Anxiety problem	Ranking

helper can offer support when you feel anxious or panicky and can help to brainstorm strategies for tackling your anxiety. Also, your helper can accompany you when you start "exposure" practices, particularly in situations you are too frightened to enter alone. Finally, involving someone else in your therapy can provide you with an extra incentive to follow through on your homework, just as having a buddy can give you that extra bit of motivation to get yourself to exercise.

There are number of characteristics that make a good helper. If you decide to involve someone else in your therapy, here are some qualities you should look for:

+ Someone you can trust, and with whom you feel comfortable discussing the details of your anxiety problem
+ Someone who is empathic and understanding
+ Someone who is willing to become familiar with the procedures used in this treatment and to read relevant parts of this book, particularly Chapter 14
+ Someone who will understand that *you* are in charge of your therapy and that his or her role is to be supportive and encouraging, and not to force you to do anything that you have not agreed to do
+ Someone who will not become angry or frustrated if you are unable to complete a particular practice, or if you become anxious during a practice

Depending on your relationship with your helper, he or she will be involved to a greater or a lesser extent in your treatment. A partner or spouse may be more inclined to read this whole book and to be highly involved in your treatment. A friend or family member, on the other hand, may be less involved and may join you only on a couple of exposure practices. You may end up deciding to involve a few different helpers so that no one person feels overly inconvenienced.

Other Ways to Involve Your Family

In addition to enlisting them as helpers, there are other ways to involve family members in your treatment. If your family members ease the way for you to continue having your anxiety problem, they may need to be instructed to stop. Family members often help their loved ones avoid the situations they fear because they want them to feel comfortable. For example, family members of an individual who is afraid to enter supermarkets may do all the grocery shopping for the family. They may do all the driving when their loved one is afraid to be behind the wheel. For people who are afraid of dogs or cats, family members may check the area outside the home for dogs and cats before their loved one leaves the house.

Although your family members and friends may have your best interests at heart when they try to protect you from feeling frightened, helping you to avoid the things you fear may make it more difficult for you to overcome your anxiety. And you may find it hard to give up this help—and may even create tension in the relationships by doing so—but it's an important step toward overcoming your anxiety. Of course, family members should be supportive and understanding, but there's a big difference between being supportive and enabling you to avoid the situations you fear.

Seeking Professional Help

There is evidence that self-help books like this one can be useful for treating certain anxiety problems even without the help of a professional therapist. Other people need a friend, a relative, or a therapist to check in on them from time to time. In fact, self-help treatments for anxiety are most effective when combined with occasional brief visits with a professional to check on progress and make sure that the treatment is on track. Others benefit most from seeing a professional and using self-help materials as a supplement to the therapy. In this section, we'll help you decide whether to seek professional help and how to select a professional who will provide the most help.

Deciding Whether to Seek Professional Help

First of all, don't feel stuck with any decision you make about whether to seek professional help. You may decide to begin treatment without the help of a therapist, but you can always change your mind if it turns out that you need extra support or guidance. Here are three factors to consider as you decide whether to hire the services of a professional.

Severity of Your Anxiety

Generally, the more severe your anxiety problem, the more likely you are to benefit from therapy with a professional, as opposed to an exclusively self-help approach. If you have multiple anxiety problems or if they are very impairing or distressing, you may want to try working with a professional in addition to using this book.

The Way You Prefer to Get Things Done

If you generally prefer to work collaboratively, then working with a therapist may be a good option, in addition to using this book. A therapist can help keep you motivated, join you for practices, provide emotional support, and answer your questions along the way. On the other hand, if you like to work independently, are a self-starter, and are able to stick to a schedule without the support of others, then working on your own may be fine.

Medication Treatment

If you would like to start or continue medication as part of your treatment, you'll need the help of a prescribing professional. All too many people "self-medicate" with drugs or alcohol. If this describes you, you may be well advised to talk to someone about pharmaceutical treatments.

How to Choose Professional Help

A first step in finding professional help is to decide what type of treatment you're seeking. Medication? Psychotherapy? A combination of the two? Some other approach? Next, consider the availability of various treatment options. In big cities, you may have the luxury of being able to choose among a large number of mental health practitioners who have experience in treating anxiety using a wide range of methods. You may even have one or more clinics in your city that specialize in treating anxiety disorders. On the other hand, you may live in a community where there are few choices available. Regardless, knowing what your options are will help you make an informed decision.

Cost of treatment is a third consideration. Make sure you know what your insurance plan will cover. And don't forget to consider both the short-term and long-term costs of treatment. Although medication treatments may cost less in the short term, over the long term the cost can add up, whereas cognitive-behavioral therapy (CBT) is often less expensive over time. This is because medication use generally continues for a much longer period (several years) compared to cognitive-behavioral treatments, which typically last only a few months.

Keep in mind that some universities have sliding-scale clinics in their psychology departments where you can receive CBT from a trainee who is supervised by a licensed psychologist. There may also be opportunities to receive treatment in the context of a research study for a reduced fee or even at no charge.

Regardless of which approach you choose, find a professional who is experienced in treating anxiety disorders using methods that have been shown to be effective. In mental health care, not all therapies are equivalent. Many practitioners use methods that are not necessarily proven to be helpful for particular problems. Be informed about what methods are most likely to be useful. It's also a good idea to interview your prospective therapist to make sure that he or she can offer what you're looking for. Examples of questions to ask include:

- ✦ What experience do you have in treating anxiety disorders? (Look for someone with experience.)
- ✦ What are your professional credentials? (Look for someone who has formal credentials, such as a psychologist, psychiatrist, social worker, or other mental health professional.)
- ✦ What sorts of approaches do you use to treat anxiety disorders? (Look for someone who uses exposure-based strategies, behavior therapy, cognitive therapy, CBT, medications, or combinations of these approaches.)

There are a number of ways to find an experienced therapist. You can contact a reputable professional association that provides referrals to members who specialize in treating anxiety disorders, such as the Anxiety Disorders Association of America (*www.adaa.org*). Many (but not all) professional members of this association have expertise in treating anxiety disorders with CBT, medications, or combinations of these approaches. There are also organizations that specialize in particular types of anxiety problems, such as the Obsessive Compulsive Foundation (*www.ocfoundation.org*), and professional associations that specialize in particular types of treatment, such as the Association for Behavioral and Cognitive Therapies (*www.abct.org*). More information on these associations, as well as other resources, are provided in the Appendix.

Other ways of finding professional help include speaking with your family doctor, visiting a local mental health clinic (especially one that specializes in anxiety disorders, if one is available in your community), and talking to people you know (health care professionals, friends, coworkers, family members) who might be aware of available options. Some communities publish guides to accessing local mental health services, including lists of practitioners in the area. There may also be information about services in your community on the Internet.

Finally, a number of programs in the United States offer intensive treatments for anxiety problems (several are listed in the Appendix). These programs typically occur over a short period (for example, 3 weeks) and are offered either on an inpatient basis or as day treatment (with daily outpatient appointments). Because these intensive programs last only a few weeks, they are often a convenient option for people who are willing to travel to get help.

Make sure you find a therapist with whom you feel comfortable working—someone you trust and with whom you can share personal information. If you find you're not happy with your therapist after a few sessions, consider finding another one.

If you're thinking about trying medications, you will need to see a professional who can prescribe. This will often be a physician (typically a family doctor or psychiatrist). Nurse practitioners can also prescribe medications; in at least two states (Louisiana and New Mexico) some psychologists are allowed to prescribe medications. A good place to start is with your primary care physician. He or she can discuss the medication options and either prescribe the medications or recommend someone who can. See Chapter 10 for a discussion of the advantages and disadvantages of medication treatments versus other types of treatment.

Choosing among Treatment Strategies

Chapters 4 through 13 each describe specific strategies for dealing with anxiety (Chapter 14 is directed to other people in your life). Depending on the types of anxiety problems you have, some of these approaches may be more relevant than others. Table 3.2 provides a list of the strategies discussed in each of these chapters and some guidelines about what sorts of problems they are most suited for.

What's Worked in the Past and What Hasn't?

Have you had treatment for your anxiety in the past? If so, think about what worked and what didn't. If a particular approach (for example, exposure, cognitive therapy, a medication) was useful in the past, consider trying it again. If a particular approach was not effective in the past, try something else this time. But consider whether unsuccessful

table 3.2. **Choosing among Various Treatment Approaches**

What is it?	Who should use it?
Cognitive strategies (Chapter 4) involve changing unrealistic, anxiety-provoking thoughts into more balanced, realistic thoughts.	These strategies are potentially useful for all anxiety-based problems, although they are used less often with very focused fears and phobias (for example, animal phobias, blood phobias), where exposure is the treatment of choice.
Exposure to fear triggers (Chapter 5) involves confronting feared situations, objects, thoughts, memories, images, feelings, and sensations, instead of avoiding them.	Exposure to fear triggers is important for anyone who fears or avoids particular external objects and situations, as well as internal experiences, such as thoughts and feelings. This chapter also discusses strategies for eliminating safety behaviors that contribute to your anxiety. Chapter 5 provides an introduction to exposure, and should be read before reading Chapters 6, 7, or 8, which focus on particular types of exposure.
Exposure to feared situations (Chapter 6) involves entering feared situations and confronting feared objects and activities.	These strategies are very important for anyone who fears and avoids objects, places, situations, or activities, such as animals, driving, social situations, being alone, touching contaminated objects, flying, and just about any other situation that you may fear. All the anxiety disorders are associated with some amount of situational fear. The more you have been avoiding encountering particular objects or situations, the more important it is to include exposure as part of your treatment.
Exposure to feared thoughts, memories, images, and urges (Chapter 7) involves repeatedly bringing on frightening thoughts, images, or impulses until they are no longer frightening.	These strategies are useful for people who are frightened by their own thoughts, memories, images, and urges, or who worry that these experiences may be dangerous in some way. Examples include people who are afraid to allow themselves to remember a traumatic event, people who worry that they may lose control or go crazy if they allow themselves to experience an anxiety-provoking thought or image, people who worry that they may act on their unwanted impulses (often the case in OCD), and people with height phobias who worry they will be drawn to the edge of a high place and jump.

(cont.)

table 3.2 *(cont.)*

What is it?	Who should use it?
Exposure to feared feelings and sensations (Chapter 8) involves exercises (for example, spinning, overbreathing, aerobic exercise) designed to bring on feared sensations repeatedly until they are no longer frightening.	These strategies are useful for people who are afraid of experiencing certain physical feelings and sensations. Examples include people who are afraid of a racing heart, who fear the consequences of dizziness, or who worry about feeling breathless. Fear of physical symptoms may occur broadly (for example, a person who fears feeling dizzy whenever it happens) or only in certain situations (for example, a person who fears feeling dizzy only when driving).
Relaxation-, meditation-, and acceptance-based strategies (Chapter 9) involve learning to relax the muscles of the body, breathe more slowly, and accept anxiety feelings rather than fight them.	Relaxation-based strategies are most useful for people who experience significant generalized anxiety, worry, and stress in their lives. They are less useful for people whose fear is tied to specific situations, such as driving, spiders, or public speaking. Meditation- and acceptance-based strategies have not been studied extensively in anxiety disorders, but preliminary evidence suggests that they may be useful for generalized anxiety and worry.
Medications and herbal remedies (Chapter 10)	Medication treatments are potentially useful for most of the anxiety disorders, with the exception of certain specific phobias such as animal phobia and blood phobias. Regardless of whether you decide to use medications as part of your treatment, it is worth reviewing Chapter 10.
Lifestyle changes (for example, diet, exercise, sleep, drug and alcohol use) (Chapter 11)	There is not much research on the relationship between living a healthy lifestyle and anxiety disorders. What we do know suggests that having a healthy lifestyle can only improve your emotional well-being.
Dealing with treatment obstacles (Chapter 12)	Regardless of which type of anxiety problems you are experiencing, this chapter is worth reviewing. In fact, you should skim it after completing this chapter, and then return to it if you notice any treatment obstacles along the way.
Preventing your anxiety from returning (Chapter 13)	Regardless of which type of anxiety problems you are experiencing, you should review the material in Chapter 13. Strategies for preventing relapse are important for staying well.

past treatments didn't work for a reason (for example, stopping a medication too soon, taking a medication at a lower-than-recommended dosage, not completing homework, and so on). If you think you may be able to do things differently this time around, it may be worth trying a past treatment again, even if it was not totally successful.

Developing a Comprehensive Treatment Plan

Your treatment plan should include strategies for dealing with the most important aspects of your anxiety. Strategies are organized in this book in the same order that you should introduce them into your own therapy. The specific techniques you use will depend on your unique anxiety profile.

Start with the cognitive strategies described in Chapter 4. After a couple of weeks of practice in challenging your thoughts, introduce exposure-based strategies, as described in Chapters 5 through 8. Use situational exposure (Chapter 6) to deal with fear and avoidance of external objects and situations. Use cognitive or imaginal exposure (Chapter 7) if you are frightened of your thoughts, images, or impulses. Use symptom exposure (Chapter 8) if you are afraid of the physical sensations associated with anxiety.

Depending on the focus of your fear, not all three types of exposure will necessarily be needed. And once you introduce exposure into your therapy, you should continue to use the cognitive strategies as well. In addition, while working on your exposure practices, it's important to begin to reduce or eliminate safety behaviors, as described in Chapter 8.

Strategies based on relaxation, meditation, or acceptance (Chapter 9) can be integrated into your therapy either after you have been practicing exposure or earlier in the treatment. For most anxiety problems, it won't be necessary to use the relaxation-, meditation-, and acceptance-based strategies at all—exposure and cognitive strategies are quite powerful on their own. But problems such as generalized anxiety, worry, and stress management may respond well to the techniques described in Chapter 9, either as an alternative to the other approaches discussed in this book or as part of a comprehensive treatment plan.

For most people, medications (Chapter 10) should be considered only if the other strategies are not effective on their own. That's because medication treatments for anxiety disorders are generally associated with higher rates of relapse following the end of treatment than are cognitive and behavioral approaches. Nevertheless, if CBT is unavailable in your community or is not effective for your symptoms, or if you have a strong preference for medications, drug treatments are likely to be effective. They can be used right from the start of treatment or added later, after CBT has been given a chance to work.

The lifestyle changes described in Chapter 11 should be integrated into treatment as soon as possible. If you think you'll find them easy to make, do it right from the start. If the changes are likely to be a challenge, try leaving them until later in your treatment. If you try to work on too many different issues at once, chances are that it will be difficult to devote the necessary time and energy to any of them.

As you work through the strategies described in this book, keep in mind the issues discussed in Chapter 12 on how to deal with obstacles. In fact, you may want to read that chapter quickly even before you begin working on the material in Chapters 4 through 11. As you encounter obstacles or challenges along the way, refer back to it. Finally, your treatment should end with attention to strategies for preventing relapse and return of symptoms, as described in Chapter 13.

Based on what you have read in this chapter, complete Form 3.5 by checking off how important you think the various strategies are likely to be in your own treatment. You can always revise your responses as you learn more about these strategies throughout this workbook.

That completes your preparation for the program! Now let's try some proven strategies for freeing you from the clutches of your anxiety.

form 3.5	**Rating the Importance of Major Treatment Strategies**		
Strategy	**Very important**	**Somewhat important**	**Not at all important**
Cognitive strategies	❑	❑	❑
Exposure to feared situations	❑	❑	❑
Exposure to feared thoughts, memories, images, and urges	❑	❑	❑
Exposure to feared feelings and sensations	❑	❑	❑
Eliminating safety behaviors and compulsions	❑	❑	❑
Relaxation-, meditation-, and acceptance-based strategies	❑	❑	❑
Medications and herbal remedies	❑	❑	❑
Lifestyle changes	❑	❑	❑
Dealing with treatment obstacles	❑	❑	❑
Preventing your anxiety from returning	❑	❑	❑

PART II

The Program

4

Changing Your Anxious Thinking

Anxious thoughts keep worry and fear alive. If you think the plane is going to crash, you're going to feel on edge during the entire flight. The strategies in this chapter help you combat excessive worry, panic attacks, and anxiety triggered by all sorts of situations and experiences, including external fears (spiders, a stuck elevator, going to the mall, losing your job), as well as internal ones (a pounding heart, memories of a trauma, an inexplicable urge to hurt your baby).

Almost all types of anxiety and fear are going to bring with them thoughts of threat and danger. And there are certainly situations in which anxiety is entirely appropriate, as when a loved one is in the hospital. It's only when these emotions grow out of proportion to the actual danger or threat that they cause a problem, interfering with your social life, your business obligations, taking care of your kids, and many other aspects of your life. We recommend that you work through this chapter even if your anxiety is of appropriate limits. You may find that even if you have good reasons to be anxious, some of your provoking thoughts may be based on exaggerated beliefs about the true risks.

The Relationship between Thoughts and Feelings

Sita was running about 30 minutes late for a routine checkup at her family doctor's office. She had left home with enough time to get to the appointment, but traffic was backed up because of an accident. Sita had left her cell phone at home, so she had no way to reach the doctor's office to let them know. What emotions do you think Sita might have been experiencing as she sat in traffic?

There's no one right answer. Different people respond to identical situations in different ways, and those responses are translated into emotions. Our beliefs, predictions, assumptions, and thoughts all influence how we feel from moment to moment. So what Sita feels as she sits in traffic is influenced by how she interprets the situation. Here are some examples of thoughts that might trigger various emotions for her:

"I'm going to be late and my doctor will be very angry." → **Anxiety**

"Those idiots should pull over so we can all get by!!!" → **Anger**

"I should have anticipated this delay. I can't do anything right!" → **Sadness**

"I was dreading this appointment—it's great to have an excuse to miss it!" → **Relief**

"This is not a big deal. I can just rebook the appointment if my doctor can't see me." → **Calmness**

Note how each interpretation or prediction leads to a very different emotional state. Also, notice that one of Sita's predictions is that her doctor will be angry. But that's just one of many possible reactions. What emotions do you think Sita's doctor might have been experiencing while waiting for Sita to arrive? Well, just as Sita's emotions are determined by her thoughts, her doctor's emotional response would likely be influenced by his thoughts about Sita's delay. Here are some examples of emotions that Sita's doctor might have experienced, and the thoughts that might have led to each of these emotions:

"I wonder if Sita is hurt or in some sort of trouble. She never misses an appointment!" → **Anxiety**

"Where the heck is she? This is costing me money!" → **Anger**

"Maybe Sita stood me up because she knows I'm not a very good doctor." → **Sadness**

"I'm running so far behind schedule today. With Sita not showing up, I may have a chance to catch up!" → **Relief**

"I'm sure Sita is late for a good reason. I'll just book her for another visit." → **Calmness**

Notice again how particular emotions are associated with particular types of thoughts. *Anxiety* is associated with interpretations involving themes of threat and danger. *Anger* can also occur when we view a situation as threatening (for example, if someone hurts our feelings), but anger and frustration can be triggered as well when we are prevented from reaching a goal (for example, sitting in bad traffic, stuck on the runway and missing our flight connection). Feelings of *sadness* and depression often occur when we have experienced some sort of loss (for example, a demotion on the job, the breakup of a relationship) or when we experience thoughts involving themes of hopelessness (for example, "I will never find a partner"). Positive feelings of *relief* occur when a potential threat or danger is removed (for example, after finding out that a loved one has returned safely from a war zone), and general feelings of *calmness* occur in response to neutral or pleasant thoughts.

Pay attention to the relationship between your thoughts and your feelings. When you learn to change your anxious thinking, you'll be reducing your levels of anxiety and fear.

The Role of Unconscious Thoughts

At this point, you may be thinking, "Sometimes I get anxious and I don't really know why." There's no question that the interpretations that trigger anxiety and fear can occur outside of our awareness. In fact, the parts of the brain that process fear (located in an area known as the "limbic system") are quite primitive. So although anxiety-provoking thoughts can trigger anxiety and fear, these emotions can also occur in response to unconscious interpretations regarding threat and danger. Even though you may experience anxiety or fear without understanding what triggered it, you can assume that in most cases your brain is interpreting your experiences as dangerous in some way. After all, fear and anxiety are the body's natural responses to perceived threat.

There are lots of examples of how we process information unconsciously. In his best-selling book *Blink,* Malcolm Gladwell provides a fascinating review of research demonstrating that quick, intuitive thinking—the kind that occurs in the "blink of an eye" (that is, unconscious information processing)—is very important in the process of making decisions, particularly in situations and during activities that are overlearned and very familiar to us.

For example, an experienced driver can safely negotiate traffic even though he or she may be consciously thinking about things other than the road. Similarly, if a bear were to jump out in front of you while you were hiking in the woods, you would need to make a split-second decision about the best way to protect yourself—there would be no time for conscious thought, which occurs much more slowly than the quick sorts of decisions we can make outside of our awareness. The sort of information processing that takes place in the limbic system allows your body to react very quickly so you can deal with situations immediately, long before conscious thought has a chance to kick in.

That's where quick thinking is helpful. With any luck, you would use it to escape the bear. Intuition, unconscious decision making, and other forms of thinking outside of awareness can also get us into trouble, however. When you've experienced a particular anxiety problem for a long time, it may become second nature to appraise even safe situations as dangerous. These evaluations may occur outside of awareness, and you may then be afraid when there's no realistic threat.

It is just this sort of response that this chapter will help you to change. The strategies in this chapter are designed to help you (1) to become more aware of your anxiety-provoking thoughts, beliefs, and interpretations; (2) to consider new ways of understanding the situations you fear; and (3) to select more realistic and balanced interpretations and predictions, when possible.

The Role of Biased Attention and Memory

If our anxiety stems from negative thinking, why doesn't anxiety naturally decrease over time as we encounter the situations we fear and see that our anxiety-provoking thoughts don't come to pass? One reason is that we often avoid the situations and experiences we fear, so we never have a chance to learn that we needn't fear them. (We'll return to this issue in the next chapter.) Another reason is that we often *ignore* information that doesn't fit with our views in favor of information that does.

Not only do we seek out and pay close *attention* to information that is consistent with our views, but we're also more likely to *remember* such information. In other words, what we see in the world and what we remember about it are not necessarily completely consistent with reality. Rather, our experiences are biased: they're influenced by our emotions and our expectations. If you're feeling sad, for example, you may dwell on sad things that have happened in your life (such as the loss of a relationship or a job) and interpret current situations more negatively. Similarly, if you're angry at your best friend, you may be more likely to interpret his or her late arrival for dinner as a sign of disrespect than you would at a time when you had kindly thoughts toward your friend.

The same holds true for anxiety. People who are anxious are more likely to pay attention to (and remember) information that is consistent with their anxiety-provoking beliefs than information that disconfirms these beliefs. Think about it:

+ If you fear spiders, you'll be the first to spot a spider in a room (perhaps because you are unconsciously "looking" for spiders).
+ When you fear flying, you may remember every detail concerning a plane crash reported in the news years earlier, but pay little attention to the millions of planes that take off and land safely each year.
+ People with panic attacks who anxiously anticipate a racing heart often scan their bodies for unusual heart sensations. Research has shown that they can also count their heartbeats more accurately than people who are not afraid of a racing heart.

So, in addition to starting to notice the content of your anxiety-provoking thoughts, you should also learn to ask yourself whether you're thinking about the situations you fear in a biased way. Be patient. This is a new way of thinking. It will take some effort to consider *all* the relevant information about these situations and experiences—not just the information that confirms your scary thoughts! But it's a very important step toward your goal of unburdening yourself of your anxiety.

Types of Anxious Thinking

Anxiety-provoking thoughts usually occur in the form of a prediction that something bad will occur (though they take other forms too). In this section we'll review thoughts and experiences that can contribute to your anxiety. You'll see that these experiences are not completely distinct from one another—they overlap a bit. Understanding these types of negative thinking will be particularly valuable as you use the strategies in this chapter to change your own anxiety-provoking thoughts.

Probability Overestimations

Do you often assume that something bad is going to happen in certain situations you fear, even though you've discovered over and over again that it doesn't? For example, someone who fears flying may assume that the risk of a particular flight crashing is high. This is very common among people with anxiety problems, and it's part of a phenomenon we call *probability overestimation*. This type of thinking may also include a superstitious component in which events that have no relationship to one another are assumed to be related (for example, "The plane is more likely to crash *if I'm on it*").

When we engage in probability overestimation, we fail to rely on statistical facts and rational thinking, relying instead on our emotions, gut feelings, anecdotes, or dramatic stories. A movie like *Jaws* or a dramatic television interview with a shark attack victim can have a much more powerful effect on our fear of swimming in the ocean than would statistics on shark attacks, which make it clear that deaths due to shark attacks are extremely rare. But one look at a shark victim and facts and figures fly out the window!

Examples of probability overestimations include statements such as these:

+ "A racing heart is a sign that I'm probably having a heart attack."
+ "Dizziness means that I'm probably going to faint."
+ "I am going to get cancer."
+ "If I park in the underground parking at work, I will get assaulted."
+ "If I allow myself to think about my rape, I will go crazy or lose control."
+ "I will make a fool of myself during my presentation."
+ "Nobody would ever want to date me."
+ "I will get into a car accident."
+ "I will get sick if I touch things in public places."
+ "I will run out of money and be broke forever."
+ "My children will get hurt."
+ "The elevator will get stuck when I am on it."

Of course, all these events are possible, but that certainly doesn't mean they're probable. One goal of this chapter is to help you to start thinking about probabilities based on the *evidence* rather than on your anxiety.

Catastrophizing

Catastrophizing (also called *catastrophic thinking*) refers to the assumption that a particular outcome will be completely unmanageable if it happens. Rather than thinking about how we might cope with a particular negative event, when we catastrophize we think about how awful the imagined event would be and how we wouldn't be able to cope with it. Whereas probability overestimation refers to exaggerating the *likelihood* of an event, catastrophizing refers to exaggerating the *importance* of the event.

Here are some examples of thoughts that reflect catastrophic thinking:

- ✦ "It would be absolutely terrible to faint."
- ✦ "I won't be able to cope if I have to drive in bad traffic."
- ✦ "It would be a disaster if I were to be rejected by someone."
- ✦ "I couldn't manage if I were to panic on an airplane."
- ✦ "Getting stuck in an elevator is one of the worst things I can imagine."
- ✦ "If I lose my job, it would be a complete disaster."
- ✦ "It would ruin my day if my teenager were to get anything less than an A in school."
- ✦ "It would be terrible to be late for an appointment."

Each of these examples takes a situation that most people would find somewhat unpleasant or inconvenient and exaggerates its ill effect. The truth is that people manage situations like these all the time. Chances are that you can also manage certain situations that probably feel as though they would be unmanageable.

Rigid Rules

Rigid rules are inflexible beliefs we have about the way things *should* be (and often include words like "should" or "must"). Rules tend to be based on our own values, so it can be difficult to prove whether they're true or false. We can, however, examine whether particular rules are *helpful* (more on this later). The rules and expectations we have for how things should be often contribute to our anxiety.

Some examples of rules that may contribute to anxiety include:

- ✦ "I should never have bad thoughts about others."
- ✦ "I must hide my anxiety from others at all cost."
- ✦ "I should be able to make my anxiety go away."
- ✦ "I should never make mistakes at work."
- ✦ "I must get an A on my exam."
- ✦ "I can never be late."
- ✦ "Children should always listen to their parents."

You can probably see the interrelationships among the types of anxiety-provoking thoughts we have discussed so far. Someone with test anxiety, for instance, might mistakenly believe that he'll do poorly on an exam (probability overestimation), that it would be terrible to get less than an A on the exam (catastrophizing), and that it's always essential to do well on exams (rule). Now let's continue with some other forms of anxious thinking.

Anxiety-Provoking Assumptions

Assumptions refer to our general beliefs about the way things are. Sometimes they're correct and sometimes they're not. In we suffer from anxiety, our assumptions often exaggerate the true level of risk or danger. These anxiety-provoking assumptions may lead us to make anxiety-provoking predictions, including probability overestimations and catastrophizing. If you have an assumption that driving is very dangerous, for example, you may predict that you're likely to be in a car accident each time you get behind the wheel. Other examples of possibly false assumptions that can contribute to anxiety include:

+ "Most large dogs are prone to attacking people."
+ "There are always lots of drunk drivers on the road."
+ "I'm not smart enough to do well on my exam."
+ "It's possible to run out of air on an elevator."
+ "People can get cancer from touching things that are contaminated."
+ "People can tell when I'm anxious."
+ "It's dangerous to feel dizzy."
+ "Being anxious can lead people to go crazy or lose control."
+ "Public bathrooms can transmit diseases."
+ "Most people don't experience anxiety."

Negative Core Beliefs

A *core belief* is one that is deeply held and quite broad, as opposed to being focused on a specific situation. Core beliefs, which often begin in childhood, color the way we view most situations. When the content of core beliefs is negative, they can contribute to feelings of anxiety and depression, as well as to other unpleasant emotions. For example, a person who has the core belief "I am incompetent" might constantly be anxious about looking stupid in front of others, about making mistakes, or about terrible things happening as a result of his or her incompetence (such as causing serious harm to others or never finding a life partner). Core beliefs can be about oneself, about other people, or about the world. Here are some examples:

+ "The world is a dangerous place."
+ "You can't trust anyone."
+ "Things will always turn out badly."
+ "I am a failure."
+ "I am defective."
+ "I am unlovable."

The general negative core belief doesn't necessarily have to be eradicated—often it's enough to work on the beliefs that arise in specific situations (for example, the car is going to crash) and ignore the question of whether more deeply held beliefs are in play. In other cases, spending some time working on your core beliefs can be helpful. This is particularly true for people who are depressed or who have experienced anxiety for a long time in a wide range of situations.

Anxiety-Provoking Impulses

Anxiety problems are sometimes associated with frightening impulses. People with obsessive–compulsive disorder (OCD) may worry that they'll do something terrible (for example, push someone into traffic, sexually abuse a child, shout something embarrassing in public), even though they have no desire to do these things and have never acted on these impulses. This is very different from people who think about harming others and actually want to do so, and who even act on the urges (such as someone who harms other people or who fantasizes about sexually abusing children).

Phobias are also sometimes associated with irrational impulses that are scary, though not dangerous. For example, someone who fears driving may feel as though he or she might be "pulled" off the road or off a bridge by an overwhelming impulse. People with a fear of heights sometimes describe an urge to jump from a high place (this is different from someone who is suicidal and has thoughts about jumping).

Of course, our anxiety problems wouldn't make us do these things. For example, OCD doesn't lead people to act on their violent thoughts, and people with height phobias don't jump from high places. These impulses are actually just examples of probability overestimations. If we have these sorts of thoughts, we predict that we're going to act on our impulses, even though the chances of actually doing so are almost zero.

Anxiety-Provoking Imagery

Normally, when we use the term *thought,* we mean what goes on when we talk to ourselves. But our thoughts can also take place through imagery. For example, rather than *thinking* "Wow, that was a beautiful painting in the museum," you might *imagine* the artwork in your mind's eye. This can happen with other senses as well. We can hum a song in our heads or imagine another person's voice talking while we're daydreaming about a past conversation.

Some people describe their anxiety-provoking predictions in the form of images. For example, rather than *thinking about* a past trauma (like a serious accident at work), a person with posttraumatic stress disorder (PTSD) may have *vivid images* of the trauma. The images may be so vivid, in fact, that it feels as thought the trauma is happening again (images of a past trauma that feel almost real are called *flashbacks*). For others, imagery is not so vivid, but may still trigger anxiety. Someone who fears socializing, for example, may have images of going to a party and being laughed at or criticized. As you work through this chapter, practice changing your anxiety-provoking imagery in addition to your anxious thinking.

Strategies for Changing Anxious Thinking

Now you should have a basic understanding of the different kinds of anxious thinking that contribute to your anxiety problems. But before you can start working on changing your thoughts, you need to change the way you *think* about your thoughts. Most of us assume our beliefs are true. Of course, it's impossible for everyone's beliefs to be true (otherwise, we would all agree about everything!).

So let's assume for a moment that some of your beliefs are not true. For the purpose of this exercise, start thinking about the beliefs that are contributing to your anxiety as *guesses* or *hypotheses*. Question these beliefs and try to evaluate them the way a scientist or a detective would look for evidence and clues before settling on a conclusion.

When you get to the point where you can accept the idea that your beliefs are not facts, changing your anxious thinking is a matter of three basic steps:

1. Becoming aware of your anxious beliefs, assumptions, and predictions
2. Considering alternative possible beliefs, assumptions, and predictions
3. Evaluating the evidence regarding your anxious beliefs, assumptions, and predictions, as well as the alternative beliefs you generated, and choosing a more realistic way of understanding the situation

Becoming Aware of Your Anxious Beliefs, Assumptions, and Predictions

In Chapter 2, you began the process of identifying your anxiety-provoking thoughts. Go back to the list you developed on Form 2.4 on page 48 to refresh your memory. Feel free to add to the list if you can think of any more.

Of course, making a list of your anxiety-provoking thoughts is just the first step. Now, whenever you experience feelings of anxiety or fear, ask yourself what you're thinking in that moment. Try to identify specific predictions that may be contributing to your discomfort and write them down. This process of monitoring your thoughts should continue throughout the time you're working on overcoming your anxiety. Below are some examples of questions you can ask yourself to help figure out what you're thinking. Questions like these are particularly useful for identifying probability overestimations, catastrophic thoughts, and anxiety-provoking impulses and images. They include general questions (particularly the first three), as well as those that are relevant to specific types of anxiety:

+ "What am I afraid will happen?"
+ "What am I predicting will occur?"
+ "What am I imagining will occur?"
+ "What am I afraid will happen if I have a panic attack in a movie theater [panic disorder]?"
+ "What will happen if I encounter a dog [dog phobia]?"
+ "As I sit here worrying about my children, are there images that come to mind about what might happen to them [generalized anxiety and worry]?"
+ "What will it mean about me if people don't like my presentation [public-speaking anxiety]?"

✦ "What will happen if I sit on a toilet seat in a public bathroom [fear of germs]?"

✦ "What do I think will happen to me if I drive on the highway [fear of driving]?"

✦ "What will happen if I get a thought about hurting another person [obsessive-compulsive, aggressive impulses]?"

✦ "What do I think will occur if I think about my past trauma [posttraumatic stress]?"

Identifying your rules and assumptions can be challenging because, as we discussed, they often occur outside of our awareness. The first step is recognizing that rules and assumptions are *not* always facts; they're just beliefs.

So how can you identify your own rules and assumptions? One way is to ask yourself, when you're feeling anxious or making anxious predictions, whether there might be any underlying rules or assumptions influencing your anxiety. For example, if you continually find yourself predicting that you're going to make a fool of yourself in front of others, is it possible that you believe in the utmost importance of always making a good impression on others (a rule)? Or, if you're predicting that you are about to faint because you feel dizzy, perhaps you have a belief that dizziness leads to fainting (an assumption).

Core beliefs are perhaps the most difficult thoughts to make ourselves aware of. One strategy for identifying core beliefs is the downward-arrow technique. Essentially, this involves repeatedly asking questions to identify the deeper meaning of your anxiety-provoking predictions. Here's an example of how a therapist might use the downward-arrow technique with a person named Brian who suffers from social anxiety:

Brian: I'm very worried about a meeting I have tomorrow. My boss is going to ask me to speak in front of the group.

Therapist: What are you worried might happen?

Brian: I'm afraid that I won't know what to say or that I may say something wrong.

Therapist: Why would that be a problem?

Brian: People will notice my mistakes.

Therapist: So what?

Brian: If they notice my mistakes, they'll think I'm stupid or incompetent.

Therapist: Why would that be a problem?

Brian: I guess that would mean that I really am incompetent.

Therapist: Do you think you are incompetent?

Brian: I guess part of me does think that.

In this example, Brian and his therapist identified a possible core belief that may contribute to his anxiety: "I am incompetent."

Writing Down Your Anxious Thoughts

When you experience anxiety, record your thoughts in the third column of an Anxiety Thought Record (see Form 4.1). This form will also be used for challenging these thoughts. More details on how to use this form are provided later in this chapter.

Considering Possible Alternative Beliefs, Assumptions, and Predictions

Another way to determine whether your beliefs are accurate is to take a broader perspective by considering other possible ways of thinking about the situation. For every anxiety-provoking thought, prediction, or interpretation, there are usually several possible alternative predictions and various different ways of understanding the situation. Table 4.1 provides a number of examples.

Stepping into Somebody Else's Shoes

If you have difficulty coming up with alternative beliefs when you're feeling anxious, another strategy is to ask yourself how someone who doesn't have an anxiety problem might interpret the situation. You can even imagine someone in particular, like a close friend, partner, or relative (for example, "How would my best friend, who is comfortable in social situations, be thinking about this party that I'm so anxious about attending?"). Chances are that this strategy will help you to think of good alternatives. Remember that your natural tendency is to think thoughts that are consistent with your anxiety. It will take conscious effort to generate different interpretations, beliefs, and predictions from the ones you've automatically had for years. But you will succeed if you stick with it.

Recording Alternative Beliefs

The fourth column of the Anxiety Thought Record (Form 4.1) provides space to record alternative beliefs.

Evaluating the Evidence and Selecting a Realistic Conclusion

Simply making a list of alternative beliefs and interpretations should help to decrease your anxiety because it will show you that your anxious thoughts are just one way of thinking about the situations you fear. Next, we take the process a step further by evaluating the evidence for and against your anxious thoughts, as well as for the alternative thoughts that you generated. This process is sometimes referred to as *challenging* your anxious thinking.

A number of different strategies can be used to challenge your anxious thoughts, including educating yourself about the situations you fear, using rational thinking to change your beliefs, and conducting experiments to test out the accuracy of your beliefs, predictions, and assumptions. In the following sections, we consider each of these approaches and discuss strategies for changing rigid rules and core beliefs.

form 4.1

Anxiety Thought Record

Day and time	Situation	Anxiety-provoking thoughts and predictions	Anxiety before (0–100)	Alternative thoughts and predictions	Evidence and realistic conclusions	Anxiety after (0–100)

table 4.1. **Generating Alternative Beliefs**

Anxiety-provoking situation and thoughts	Examples of alternative beliefs and interpretations
Situation: My husband is 30 minutes late coming home from work, and he isn't answering his mobile phone. **Thought:** He has been in a serious car accident.	"He stopped somewhere on the way home from work." "He left work late." "He is stuck in traffic." "He has been in a minor fender bender." "His phone is turned off." "He is in an area with poor reception." "He left his phone at work or somewhere else." "The battery in his phone needs to be charged." "He is talking on the phone and can't take my call."
Situation: I have agreed to have lunch with some coworkers. **Thought:** I will have nothing to say or I will say stupid things. They will think I'm stupid and boring!	"Perhaps they won't think I'm boring." "Perhaps they won't think I'm stupid." "Perhaps I will be able to think of intelligent things to say."
Situation: I am riding an elevator. **Thought:** The elevator will get stuck and I will suffocate.	"The elevator may not get stuck." "Even if the elevator gets stuck, I may not suffocate."
Situation: I am having a panic attack and feeling unreal and dizzy. **Thought:** Dizziness means that I am about to go crazy or lose control.	"Dizziness can occur because I haven't eaten." "Dizziness can occur because of low blood pressure or standing up too quickly." "Dizziness can occur because of anxiety." "I may be experiencing dizziness simply because I am scanning my body, looking for feelings of dizziness (I might not notice the feeling if I wasn't looking for it)." "People don't go crazy from dizziness." "People don't lose control from dizziness."

(cont.)

table 4.1 (cont.)

Anxiety-provoking situation and thoughts	Examples of alternative beliefs and interpretations
Situation: I am walking through the mall and someone walks toward me. **Thought:** He is going to attack me or try to rob me.	"Perhaps he is just going to walk by me." "Perhaps he will ask me a question." "Perhaps he wants to tell me something." "Perhaps he is walking toward someone who is standing behind me."
Situation: An intrusive OCD thought about stabbing my wife pops into my head. **Thought:** Thinking about stabbing my wife means that I'm likely to do it.	"Having a thought is not the same as acting on the thought." "I am not going to stab my wife." "Thinking about stabbing my wife doesn't increase the likelihood of doing it."

Using the Anxiety Thought Record

As you work through the rest of this chapter, start to use the entire Anxiety Thought Record (Form 4.1) every time you feel anxious (or at least several times per week, if your anxiety episodes are too numerous to record). Table 4.2 explains how the form should be completed.

Education

You're not going to have an easy time figuring out whether your beliefs are true if there are important gaps in your knowledge about the situations you fear. One strategy for gathering evidence about the accuracy of your thoughts is to educate yourself. How you do this depends on the nature of the situations that make you anxious. Table 4.3 includes ways you can use education and information gathering to challenge anxious thoughts for all kinds of anxiety issues. Sources of information can include other people (friends, relatives, experts), books, television, and the Internet. Be sure to check multiple sources, and be careful not to rely on sources that may be biased.

Suppose you're trying to learn more about the risks of flying, for instance. Don't just check websites of the major airlines (which may underestimate the risks) or talk to others who fear flying (who may exaggerate the risks). Check out multiple sources, and as many neutral sources as possible. For example, the website for the National Safety Council provides statistics for death by various causes (*www.nsc.org/research/odds.aspx*), and shows that the odds of dying in a plane crash are much less than from many other causes, including dying from a simple fall.

Rational Thinking

Rational thinking involves trying to shift your thinking by asking yourself questions such as "Do my thoughts make sense in light of all the information I have?" and "Are there other ways to look at this situation that make more sense based on the facts?" One example of a strategy for thinking more rationally is to examine your past experiences and to use them to make more accurate predictions about the future. Consider the following discussion between Mike and his therapist:

> *Mike*: Every time I go into a public place like a restaurant or theater, I worry that I may have uncontrollable diarrhea and that I won't make it to the bathroom on time. It's easiest just to avoid these situations.
>
> *Therapist*: Do you have that thought *every* time you're out in public?
>
> *Mike*: Well, not every time. Maybe about a third of the time.

table 4.2. **How to Complete the Anxiety Thought Record**

Column	How to complete
1. Day and time	Record the date and time when your anxiety episode occurred.
2. Situation	Describe the situation that triggered your anxiety. This can be an object, activity, or experience (for example, a thought, memory, image, or physical feeling).
3. Anxiety-provoking thoughts and predictions	Record any anxiety-provoking thoughts or predictions that were on your mind. What were you afraid might happen?
4. Anxiety before (0–100)	Using a scale ranging from zero (completely calm) to 100 (completely terrified), rate your anxiety level before you started to challenge your anxious thoughts.
5. Alternative thoughts and predictions	Record some alternative beliefs and predictions to counter the thoughts listed in column 3.
6. Evidence and realistic conclusions	Using the strategies described in the remainder of this chapter, record any evidence you can think of to counter your anxiety-provoking thoughts. Based on this evidence, write down a realistic conclusion or prediction.
7. Anxiety after (0–100)	Using a scale ranging from zero (completely calm) to 100 (completely terrified), rate your anxiety level after challenging your anxious thoughts.

table 4.3. **Using Education to Challenge Anxious Thoughts**

Issue	Strategies for Gathering New Information
"I'm concerned that others will think my presentation is boring."	Collect data at the end of your presentation, and have attendees rate their satisfaction with various aspects of the presentation, including how interesting it was.
	Ask a few attendees whom you trust to provide honest feedback about your presentation.
"I believe that snakes are dangerous."	Find out whether snakes in your area are in fact dangerous and how to distinguish between the dangerous ones and the harmless ones.
	Learn about the conditions under which snakes attack and how to tell whether a snake is likely to be aggressive.
	Find out what particular snake behaviors mean (for example, What does it mean when a snake sticks out its tongue?).
"I worry that my plane will crash, especially when I hear strange noises during a flight."	Seek out statistics on the frequency of plane crashes and the conditions under which crashes tend to occur.
	Learn about the meaning of various sounds that occur on the plane.
"I worry that the elevator will get stuck and I will die of suffocation."	Seek out statistics (perhaps from a company that installs and repairs elevators) concerning how often elevators get stuck.
	Ask an expert how elevators are ventilated and whether it is possible to run out of air.
	Look for information about the frequency of elevator-related deaths.
"I'm convinced I'm going to be struck by lightning whenever there is a thunderstorm."	Learn more about thunderstorms, including how often they occur, how often people are struck by lightning, and how often people who are struck by lightning are severely injured or killed.
"I worry that my heart palpitations are a sign that I am having a heart attack."	Learn about the risks for heart disease and whether you have any of the most important risk factors.
	Arrange for a physical with your family doctor to rule out any medical problems (but don't do this over and over again—*too much* reassurance seeking can be a problem!).
	Learn about the signs and symptoms of heart disease.

Therapist: Of these times, how often have you actually had diarrhea?

Mike: Not often. Maybe just two or three times. But the way my stomach rumbles, I sure feel like it's going to happen much more often than that. Besides, even two or three times is too many times to lose control of my bowels in public!

Therapist: Have you actually had diarrhea in public, or have you made it to a bathroom in time?

Mike: Fortunately, I've always made it to the bathroom just in time. But I was lucky. Who knows what would have happened if I didn't have a bathroom nearby?

Therapist: Have you ever had the feeling that you needed a bathroom and couldn't get to one?

Mike: Actually, that's happened a few times.

Therapist: What was the outcome?

Mike: Eventually the feeling passed. I guess I didn't need the bathroom after all.

Therapist: So, of all the times you have been out in public, your feared consequence has never actually occurred. Even when you didn't have access to a bathroom, you survived without losing bowel control. What does that tell you about the next time you're in a public place?

Mike: I guess the likelihood of having uncontrollable diarrhea is not as great as I think.

Notice how the therapist repeatedly asks Mike questions to help him come to a more realistic conclusion about his feared situation. We encourage you to ask yourself questions to challenge your own anxious thinking. See Table 4.4 for some suggestions.

Decatastrophizing

Decatastrophizing, just as it sounds, is a way to combat catastrophizing—remember, that's when we exaggerate the importance of a possible event and assume that it will be absolutely terrible and completely unmanageable. Often, when we anticipate some negative event, we assume that it will be awful and that we'll be unable to cope—but we stop short of imagining what it will actually be like and just how we'll react if it were to occur. Decatastrophizing involves taking your catastrophic thoughts to this next stage, thereby taking away their power.

Decatastrophizing involves asking yourself two simple questions:

1. Realistically, what is the worst that could happen?
2. How would I cope with that?

The goal is to discover that the worst is not all that bad, and that there's an excellent chance you will be able to cope with most situations that are likely to come up in your life. Here are some examples of how decatastrophizing can be used to fight catastrophic thinking:

table 4.4. **Questioning Yourself to Challenge Anxious Beliefs**

Anxiety-provoking belief	Examples of questions to ask yourself
"I worry that I'll make a fool of myself if I go to the party."	"What has my experience been in the past? Do I normally get feedback from others that I come across as foolish at parties?" "Don't most people say something foolish from time to time?" "Is it really so important that I come across perfectly? What are some of the benefits of allowing myself to make mistakes?" "So what if some people think I look foolish?" "What advice would I give to a close friend who was having this thought?"
"A spider will crawl on me, and I won't be able to cope."	"How often do I actually see spiders?" "Of those times, how often do they crawl on me?" "Am I generally able to cope okay in stressful situations?" "Based on my past experiences with spiders, what is the worst thing that will happen?" "How long will it take to get the spider off me? Will it really matter if a spider is on me for a few seconds or less?" "Other than feeling uncomfortable, are there any negative consequences? If not, can I handle feeling uncomfortable for a few seconds?"
"When I have a headache, I worry that it may be a brain tumor."	"How often have I had headaches in the past?" "How often do other people have headaches?" "What are some of the other triggers for my headaches?" "Have any of my past headaches been caused by a tumor?" "What are all the reasons why people get headaches, other than tumors? How common are these other causes?"
"I'm convinced that I will die in a car accident every time I get into a car."	"How often have I been in a car?" "Of those times, how often have I worried about getting into an accident?" "Of those times, how often have I actually been in an accident?" "What do I know about the percentage of accidents that are fatal (based on available statistics)?"

table 4.4 *(cont.)*

Anxiety-provoking belief	Examples of questions to ask yourself
"I'm convinced that I will die in a car accident every time I get into a car." *(cont.)*	"What does this tell me about the chances of dying in a car accident the next time I go for a drive?" "What are the factors that increase the risk of a car accident (for example, drinking, speeding, talking on the phone, following too closely, not paying attention)? Do I do any of those things?"
"If I panic on a plane, I will drop dead of a heart attack."	"Is there any evidence that panic attacks cause heart attacks?" "Is there any evidence that a racing heart is dangerous? In fact, my heart races during exercise, and that's supposed to be good for the heart!" "What are all the reasons other than heart disease why hearts race (for example, arousal, exercise, anxiety, caffeine)?" "What does my past experience tell me about the likelihood of dying during a panic attack? (I have panicked many times before and not died.)" "What are the risk factors for heart attack (for example, older age, smoker, overweight, high blood pressure, high cholesterol, family history of heart disease)? Do I have many of these?"
"I will lose control if I think about how I was abused as a child."	"What do I mean by 'lose control'?" "Have I ever actually lost control before?" "Does trying not to think about the abuse work, or does it lead me to think about it even more?"
"Others will notice my anxiety symptoms (especially my shaking) and will think I'm weak or strange."	"What else might people think if they notice my shaking (for example, they might think I'm cold)?" "Are there things other than 'I'm weak or strange' that people might think about me if they notice I am anxious?" "Does it really matter if some people think I am anxious (after all, I sometimes notice other people's anxiety, and they don't seem to suffer any negative consequences as a result)?" "Do I have the right to look anxious sometimes?"

(cont.)

table 4.4 *(cont.)*

Anxiety-provoking belief	Examples of questions to ask yourself
"If I don't worry about my children, that means I'm a bad mother."	"Do children with worried mothers generally grow up healthier?" "Are there any negative consequences for me or my children of worrying about them too much?" "What would happen if I worried about my children even a bit less often?" "What advice would I give to a close friend who was having this thought?"
"It's important for everyone to like me."	"What would happen if someone didn't like me (for example, a cashier in a store, a stranger on the street, a coworker)?" "Is it possible for everyone to like me?" "Can I think of a person I know whom *everybody* likes?" "Can I think of a person I know whom *nobody* likes?" "Isn't it true that the very things that will make me likeable to some people will make me less likeable to others?"
"Everything must be neat and tidy. It's important that everything be in its place. If I let even a few things get out of place, everything will turn to chaos."	"Do I have any evidence that letting a few things go will lead to chaos?" "What will happen if a few things are out of order?" "Could I survive feeling uncomfortable for a while because a few items at home are out of place?"

Catastrophic thought: "It would be awful to faint during a panic attack."

Decatastrophizing: "What would actually happen if I fainted? Well, I probably would be unconscious for a few seconds and would then regain consciousness. People would probably help me. It would be a bit embarrassing, but that feeling would pass. I guess it wouldn't be the end of the world."

Catastrophic thought: "It would be terrible if I said something stupid in front of others."

Decatastrophizing: "So what if I say something stupid? People say stupid things all the time, and often they don't even seem to care. If I were to say something stupid, a few people might notice, and others might not. Some people might comment on it, and that would be the end of it. It probably wouldn't matter a few minutes

	later, and it certainly wouldn't matter the next day or the next week."
Catastrophic thought:	"It would be awful if my car isn't fixed by the time the mechanic said it would be ready."
Decatastrophizing:	"What would happen if my car isn't ready? Why would that be such a problem? Could I cope with it? Well, if it's not ready, it would be inconvenient. I would have to get a ride with someone else or take public transportation to work. I could live with that for a few more days if I had to."
Catastrophic thought:	"It's terrible to have an intrusive, inappropriate sexual or aggressive thought about another person."
Decatastrophizing:	"What is the consequence of having such a thought? Thoughts don't equal actions. Also, the more I try to fight my thoughts, the worse they get. I should just let my thoughts happen. The worst that will occur is that I'll feel uncomfortable. That would be okay. Everyone has inappropriate thoughts sometimes, even though they may not talk about them."
Catastrophic thought:	"I think I would want to kill myself if I lost my job."
Decatastrophizing:	"How could I cope with losing my job? It would be difficult, but I could live off my credit cards, or with help from relatives, until I found a new job. I could apply for all sorts of positions, or I could even go back to school. I recently read that the typical American changes jobs every 3½ years. If others are able to find a new job that often, then I should be able to find one as well."

Experiments

Earlier in this chapter, we mentioned that changing your anxious thoughts involved thinking like a scientist. So, how do scientists make discoveries? They conduct experiments. If a researcher believes that treating high blood pressure with changes in diet and exercise is likely to be more effective than a standard medication treatment, she might test out this hypothesis by conducting an experiment. She might take a large group of people with high blood pressure and give half of them medication and the other half instructions to change their diet and exercise regimes. If the treatment involving changes to diet and exercise works best, that's a sign that the researcher's hypothesis may be correct. It would also be important to see if the results could be repeated over several studies by several different researchers, since the results of any one study may be due to chance or to problems with how the study is designed.

Experiments can also be used to test out your own anxiety-provoking predictions. For example, Lara's panic attacks tended to be triggered by any activity that made her heart race, like exercise or sex. She was convinced that if she didn't stop exercising or having sex when she started to feel panicky, she would collapse from a heart attack. So she always rested when she noticed her panicky feelings coming on. She eventually stopped exercising or having sex altogether. Lara believed that sitting down when she felt panicky was the only way to prevent a heart attack and perhaps to save her life. When her therapist asked her to come up with an alternative, nonanxious belief, she acknowledged that another interpretation would be that her panic attacks and racing heart are not dangerous, and that sitting down has nothing to do with the fact that she doesn't die during her attacks.

Can you think of an experiment that could be designed to test out which of these two beliefs is correct? Well, one option is for Lara to exercise and then not sit down when she starts to feel panicky. As long as she is physically healthy, which her family doctor has confirmed, there would be little to no risk in trying an experiment like this, and it could show Lara that she doesn't need to rest when she feels panicky during exercise.

Similar experiments can be designed to test out a whole range of anxious beliefs. Table 4.5 provides examples of specific predictions that would be likely to lead to anxiety, along with experiments that could be used to test out each prediction. Experiments do require that you take some minor risks, but they'll be no greater than the types of risks most people take every day.

Now you're ready to plan some of your own experiments. Use the Experiment Form (Form 4.2) to plan an experiment and record your results. In the first column, record an anxiety-provoking thought or prediction. In the second column, list one or more alternative (non-anxiety-provoking) thoughts or predictions. In the third column, describe the experiment you will do to test out whether the belief recorded in column 1 is accurate. In the fourth column, record the outcome of your experiment. What actually occurred? What evidence did you gain? Did your prediction come true? What did you learn from the experiment? What did it tell you about the accuracy of your original prediction? Now record a more accurate thought, based on the results of your experiment.

Make it a point to conduct a certain number of experiments a week and complete an Experiment Form each time.

Changing Rigid Rules

Rigid rules are often hard to change because (1) they're difficult to prove or disprove, and (2) they're based on personal values, and we resist changing our values because we don't want to compromise our integrity.

It's up to you to decide which rules and values are worth changing. It's also up to you to decide how much to change a particular rule or value. For example, if you believe that "It's *always* important to make a good impression on others," you wouldn't want to replace that rule with something like "It's *never* important to make a good impression on others." Rather, ask yourself questions that will help you become more flexible with respect to this rule. You might ask whether it's even possible to make a good impression on other people all the time. What are the costs of always having to look good in front of others? Are the costs worth it? Are there some situations in which the consequences of making a bad impression are acceptable? Do other people hold the same values?

table 4.5. **Using Experiments to Challenge Anxious Beliefs**

Anxiety-provoking thought	Examples of possible experiments
"I'll get sick if I don't wash my hands after being out in public."	Don't wash your hands for one day and see if you get sick.
"It would be terrible if I were to look anxious in public."	Let yourself purposely look anxious. Put an anxious look on your face, let your hands shake, and put some water on your forehead to simulate sweating. Then go out in public. Do people seem to notice? Do they seem to care? Are there any negative consequences at all, other than your feeling uncomfortable?
"I phone my husband every hour during the day because I always need to know where he is in case something terrible happens to one of us."	Try *not* calling your husband for one day. Other than feeling uncomfortable, does anything bad happen?
"If I ask others for directions, they will think I'm stupid."	Stand in a public place for an hour and ask everyone who walks by for directions. Is there any indication that most of them think you're stupid?
"If I go out on a date with a man, he will attack me."	Try going out on a date (of course, take the precautions that most people would take: make sure you know something about the person and/or have the first date in a public place, and the like). Do you get attacked?
"If I make a left turn in the car, I will get hit by another driver."	Try making lots of left turns for an hour or so, and see what happens.

By answering questions like these, you may discover that it's quite impossible to meet your own high standards, that other people don't hold the same standards, and that the costs of trying to meet your standards far outweigh the benefits. Just by loosening up your expectations and rules, you may find that your anxiety decreases.

Changing Core Beliefs

As we mentioned earlier, negative core beliefs are the most deeply held elements of anxious thinking. If you have identified one or more core beliefs that contribute to your own anxiety, try to challenge them. The strategies for changing core beliefs are similar to those for changing other types of negative thinking.

Experiment Form

Anxiety-provoking thoughts and predictions	Alternative thoughts and predictions	Experiment description	Evidence and realistic conclusions/Anxiety after completing experiment

First, identify some alternative core beliefs. If you believe that you're incompetent, for example, you might consider the alternative belief that you're competent. When examining labels such as "competent" and "incompetent," try to define your terms. What does it mean to you to be considered incompetent or competent? This is the essential first step in gathering evidence to challenge your negative core beliefs.

The next step is to start seeking evidence. Remember, your natural tendency will be to notice information that confirms your negative core belief. Continuing with our example, if you're convinced that you're incompetent, it will be very easy to notice and remember the mistakes you make and much more difficult to notice and remember the competent things you do. Therefore, it can be useful to start keeping a Positive Data Log (see Form 4.3), a diary in which you record each time something happens that disproves your negative core belief. It's a good idea to fill this in throughout the day, and to review the information you record on a regular basis. Over time, collecting this information, along with using the other strategies in this chapter, will chip away at your negative core beliefs.

Troubleshooting

Although the strategies described in this chapter are effective tools for reducing anxiety, obstacles sometimes arise along the way. Here are some of the most common problems that may come up, along with some possible solutions.

Problem: "I can't figure out what my anxious thoughts are."

Solution: First, if you're not aware of any specific anxious thoughts (such as "If I have a panic attack, I will go crazy, lose control, or die"), try to identify whether there are some less specific thoughts that are influencing your fear (for example, "Something bad will happen, though I don't know what; I won't be able to cope with the anxiety feelings; the anxiety won't end").

Second, consider the possibility that instead of specific *thoughts*, perhaps it is anxiety-provoking *images* that contribute most to your anxiety. Are you aware of any such imagery?

Third, perhaps you're finding it difficult to identify thoughts because you're not actually anxious in the moment. Sometimes, triggering anxiety can help to make a person more aware of his or her anxiety-provoking thoughts. Try triggering your own anxiety by entering the situation you fear or imagining being in the situation. Then ask yourself again what sorts of anxiety-provoking predictions you are aware of.

If you still can't identify your anxious thoughts, don't worry. The strategies you'll learn later in the book will be useful even if you can't identify these thoughts.

Problem: "I used the cognitive strategies to challenge my anxious thoughts, but there was no change in my anxiety."

Solution: It often takes a while for the cognitive strategies to start working. At first,

Positive Data Log

Negative core belief:

Day and time	Information that disconfirms my negative core belief

they may seem superficial, obvious, or silly. With practice, however, the new nonanxious thoughts should become stronger and the anxiety-provoking thoughts should weaken. If you don't see a shift in your anxiety, consider the possibility that the thoughts you're working on are not the ones that are most closely related to your anxiety. Are there other thoughts that may be more relevant? It's possible too that there is additional evidence you haven't considered. You may need to dig deeper to find additional evidence to challenge your anxious thoughts. Someone else (who doesn't share the same thoughts) may be able to help you come up with additional evidence.

If your anxiety remains high after trying the strategies in this chapter, don't be discouraged! You'll learn many other techniques as you work your way through this book.

Problem: "Writing down my thoughts makes me more anxious because it keeps me focused on my anxiety triggers."

Solution: As you'll learn in the next chapter, repeated exposure to situations that trigger your anxiety should lead to a decrease in anxiety over the long term. Keep completing your Anxiety Thought Records and the process should get easier over time.

Problem: "I hate filling out forms. It reminds me of being in school."

Solution: Even this isn't a problem. The main purpose of the forms is to help you to think differently about the situations you fear. If you can do that better without the forms, or by using some other strategy (such as using a diary or tape-recording your responses instead of writing them down), that's fine. Another option is to simplify the forms. Maybe you'd like to develop your own Anxiety Thought Record with just two columns: one for your anxious thoughts and one for your more realistic thoughts.

But before giving up on the forms, try to complete them a few times to see if they become more helpful over time.

Problem: "When I'm feeling anxious, I'm too wound up to use the strategies in this chapter or to complete the forms."

Solution: If you know you're going to have to enter an anxiety-provoking situation, try using the strategies and completing an Anxiety Thought Record *before* entering the situation and before your anxiety has had a chance to peak. Or complete the form later, after your anxiety has decreased. This will provide you with an opportunity to work through what you might have said to yourself when your anxiety was at its peak, which should help you the next time you find yourself in the situation.

Problem: "I'm not experiencing any anxiety lately because I avoid the situations I fear. So I have nothing to record on my Anxiety Thought Record."

Solution: Well, you need something to work with. Try confronting situations that arouse at least some anxiety if you're not ready to face the biggest fears yet.

Conclusion

Anxiety is often triggered by a tendency to assume that situations are more dangerous than they really are. Sometimes these assumptions are so quick and automatic that they occur outside our awareness. When we're anxious, we also tend to give greater weight to information that confirms our anxious beliefs and to discount or ignore information that isn't consistent with these beliefs. This biased way of processing information helps keep our anxiety alive.

There are a number of types of anxious thinking, including probability overestimations, catastrophic thinking, adhering to overly rigid rules, anxiety-provoking assumptions, negative core beliefs, anxiety-provoking impulses, and anxiety-provoking imagery. Changing anxious thinking begins with viewing our thoughts as guesses about the way things may be rather than as facts. Other key steps include (1) becoming more aware of our anxious thoughts, (2) considering alternative nonanxious interpretations and predictions, and (3) evaluating the evidence for and against the available interpretations to come up with a realistic way of looking at the situation. Challenges may arise when using these strategies, but most people experience a significant drop in anxiety after learning to challenge their anxiety-provoking beliefs. With practice, you will too.

5

Eliminating the Safety Net

In 1999, Dr. David Satcher, then U.S. surgeon general, wrote perhaps the most complete review of mental health and treatment ever published. In it, he stated that the most important and critical part of treatment for anxiety is "exposure to the stimuli or situations that provoke anxiety"—in other words, facing your fears. Experts in the treatment of anxiety call this *exposure.*

In this chapter, you'll learn about the elements of planning and conducting your own exposures. Subsequent chapters will address using exposures for different kinds of anxiety problems. Chapter 6 provides important additional tips for exposures to *objects and situations* that cause you anxiety; Chapter 7 describes exposure to fearful *thoughts*; and Chapter 8 discusses exposure to fearful *sensations* in your body. In each chapter, we'll show you how to develop a step-by-step plan to begin confronting your fears, starting with the easier fears.

Exposure involves confronting the situations, objects, sensations, or thoughts that trigger your anxiety. A person with a fear of needles might practice handling needles, getting a shot at the doctor's office, or having blood drawn by a qualified professional. Don't try to confront your worst fears immediately or to face all your fears at once! Experts in the treatment of anxiety call that *flooding.* Although it can be effective, it should be done only with the help of an experienced mental heath professional. Instead, we recommend *graduated exposure,* starting with your easier fears and then, when you have gained confidence and success in overcoming those fears, gradually moving on to more difficult fears.

Exposure will probably be the most important strategy for your recovery. Unfortunately, it can also be the most difficult strategy because it requires you to do exactly what your mind has been telling you *not* to do. And it only works if you give 100%. So you have to be ready to make a commitment to it. When you are, sign the Exposure Contract, and rely on it to motivate you when you start to slip. Clip it out of this book and carry it with you or post it on the refrigerator if that helps. (Chapters 3 and 12 may also be helpful when your motivation needs a boost.)

EXPOSURE CONTRACT

I have the **CONFIDENCE, COURAGE,** and **COMMITMENT** to start confronting my fears, the easier ones today and the harder ones in the weeks to come.

_____

Signature

How Does Exposure Work?

Reading Joseph's story will help you understand how exposure works and how successful it can be. In telling his story, we've interjected some questions for you to think about.

Joseph and the Diving Board

Joseph celebrated his 12th birthday with his family and friends at the local public pool. This pool had been built for international competition, so it had a full range of diving platforms. These platforms were open only to people age 12 and older—that's exactly why Joseph wanted his birthday there. He couldn't wait because he had seen his older brother have fun jumping from the diving boards dozens of times.

Joseph eagerly climbed the ladder to the 10-foot-high platform—but then he looked down. To his young eyes, it seemed he was a mile in the air, and the water no longer seemed as if it would be soft to land in. He desperately wanted to turn around and head back down the ladder.

- If Joseph had turned around and escaped his fears, do you think he would be *more* or *less* likely to try diving again?
- How might turning around and escaping his fear make Joseph feel about himself?

Fortunately, Joseph's family and friends were in the water, encouraging him to jump. Even though he was scared, he mustered up his courage and jumped, screaming in terror the whole way down. After the splash, he felt astonished that he was still alive. His first thought was that he never wanted to do that again. But he watched the other kids having fun jumping from the diving board, and his family encouraged him to try it again. As he climbed back up, he still felt afraid, but not as much as last time, which seemed strange. He found it a little easier to jump the second time. And it wasn't as scary on the way down. The third time was even better, and so was the fourth. By the fifth time, he was racing up the ladder and letting out a shout of "*Woo-hoo!*" as he flung himself into the water.

- By confronting his fears again and again, Joseph made them gradually disappear, and he actually began to enjoy himself.
- Have you had an experience like Joseph's where you were initially scared but felt better after trying something a few times?

Joseph didn't know it, but he was doing exposure therapy. By repeatedly confronting his fear, he lost the feeling of terror when standing on the diving board. Later that day he climbed up to the 5-meter (about 15 feet) board. Was he scared? You bet! But not quite as scared as the first time he had stood on the lowest platform. After a few jumps, he lost his fear and just enjoyed himself. The same process happened a few weeks later when he tried the 7.5-meter platform.

This is graduated exposure: confronting your fears gradually, starting with easier situations and building up to harder ones as your anxiety starts to diminish.

Why Does Exposure Work?

Psychologists have studied exposure therapy since the 1960s. They have found that the more we confront something, the less we tend to react to it. Remember that really scary movie you saw a few years back? Do you think it would have been as scary if you had watched it again the next day? How about a third time? A fourth time? A tenth? It's human nature to get used to things over time, but only as long as you allow human nature the chance to get used to them, just as Joseph did.

Why does exposure work? One possibility is that it allows us to learn that our feared outcome doesn't come to pass. In the last chapter, you learned strategies for changing your anxious thoughts. But it's one thing to *tell* yourself that something bad isn't going to happen (or that it won't be as bad as you think if it does happen) and another thing entirely to *prove* it to yourself. Remember poor Joseph when he first stood on the edge of the diving platform? What do you think he was expecting to happen if he jumped? He probably thought he would feel horrible and that he might get hurt or die. What do you think he thought after he jumped the first time? Probably that it felt horrible, but that he didn't get hurt or die. What about the next time? Not so horrible, didn't get hurt or die, and a little exhilarating. Next time: "This is fun! Why was I so scared before?" He proved his anxious thoughts wrong.

Exposure has the added benefit of promoting confidence and courage. Each time you successfully confront your fears, you give yourself an extra boost of self-confidence. You tell yourself "I did it, and I can do it again." And you start to feel that you can try other things you've been avoiding. You're getting control of your anxiety—and your life! This feeling of confidence is almost addictive. The more you overcome, the more you want to push yourself further. It's just like an athlete who makes her personal best performance. She knows she can do it, she believes that she can do even better, and she wants to try even harder next time. And so will you.

form 5.1	**Exposure Plan**	
Rank order	**Situation, object, or fear trigger**	**Fear rating (0–100)**

Creating an Exposure Plan

The first step in beginning exposure is to create a list of the triggers that cause you to feel anxious. You can use the situations you listed on the forms in Chapter 2 as a start. Then, using Form 5.1, list 10 situations, objects, physical sensations, or thoughts/memories that cause you fear or discomfort or that you avoid because of your anxiety. Make sure to list some that cause less fear and some that cause more. You can break apart some triggers into easier and harder parts, such as *seeing a plastic snake* versus *seeing a real snake,* or *going to an empty supermarket* versus *going to the supermarket when it is busy.* If you're working on more than one type of fear, use different forms if that makes it easier for you. In most cases a list of 10 triggers, which includes some of your most difficult fears, is enough. But feel free to list more. Be as specific as you can in listing the trigger.

Once you've come up with about 10 triggers or objects, go back and rank them in order from 1 (the worst or most frightening trigger) to 10 (the least frightening trigger on the list). Finally, for each trigger, make a rating about how much fear or discomfort you would experience if you were to face it. Rate each situation or object from 0 (wouldn't scare you at all) to 100 (the scariest thing you can imagine).

When you're done, you may find it helpful to write out the list again, in order of difficulty, from 1 (the hardest situation or object) to 10 (the easiest situation or object). Usually it's best if the #1 trigger is something that has a fear rating of 80 to 100, and the #10 trigger has a fear rating of about 30 or 40. This will give you a ladder you can move up as you start to confront more and more difficult triggers, just as Joseph moved up to higher and higher diving platforms. Now, on Form 5.2, rewrite your list in order of difficulty.

Form 5.3 shows an example of an Exposure Plan for Miguel, a 28-year-old who works in an architectural firm. Miguel has been experiencing a lot of social anxiety and is very fearful of speaking to others, especially people in authority. He's extremely anxious about giving talks and speaking up during meetings, but he also finds himself avoiding social activities, such as playing softball, because he worries that he might mess up and everyone will laugh at him.

Marcus is also working to overcome his anxiety. He has some social fears, like Miguel, but he also becomes anxious in places where he feels unsafe, such as elevators, heights, and when driving on the freeway. He's also bothered by memories of a bad car accident a few years back. Take a look at Marcus's Exposure Plan on Form 5.4.

Carrying Out Your Exposure Plan

In the next three chapters we'll give you more specific details about how you can conduct exposures to situations or objects, physical sensations, and thoughts or memories. Please read those chapters that were identified in your treatment plan (Chapter 3) as being important for you before beginning your exposures. All exposure exercises have aspects in common that we will discuss here.

Exposure Plan in Order of Difficulty

Rank order	Situation, object, or fear trigger	Fear rating (0–100)
1		
2		
3		
4		
5		
6		
7		
8		
9		
10		

form 5.3	**Miguel's Exposure Plan**	
Rank order	**Situation, object, or fear trigger**	**Fear rating (0–100)**
1	Giving a speech at work to the managers	100
2	Performance reviews at work with my supervisor	95
3	Practice speeches with friends	90
4	Meetings with my supervisor at work	80
5	Playing softball on the company team	70
6	Playing softball on a city league team	60
7	Small talk at work with bosses or supervisors	55
8	Small talk with coworkers	50
9	Calling work clients on the telephone	40
10	Calling friends on the telephone	30

form 5.4	**Marcus's Exposure Plan**	
Rank order	**Situation, object, or fear trigger**	**Anxiety rating (0–100)**
1	Talking in front of a large group	90
2	Crowded elevators	85
3	Meeting new people	85
4	Driving on the freeway with heavy traffic	80
5	Memories of my car accident	80
6	Driving on the freeway with little traffic	60
7	Heights (over 10 feet up)	50
8	Empty elevator	50
9	Heights (5 to 10 feet up)	30
10	Crowds	20

Choosing a Good Exposure

Remember, the goal is to start with easier exposures and then work your way up to the more difficult ones when you feel ready. It may seem daunting at first, but you can do this—many others before you have successfully done it. Look over your plan. Are triggers 10 or 9 things that you could easily arrange to face? Are they exposures that would cause *some* anxiety, but not be overwhelming?

Carefully select your first exposure, then take the following few steps to ensure that you get as much benefit as possible from it.

1. Identify exactly how you're going to arrange the exposure. This is important. If you can't *arrange* to do the exposure, you can't *do* the exposure! Take some time to figure out exactly how you can make it happen. Don't leave it to chance or "wing it" and see what happens. If your exposure involves touching things in the bathroom that you fear might be covered in germs, make sure you have a private bathroom that you can use. If it involves being around snakes, check to see if your local zoo has a snake exhibit. If it involves going somewhere that reminds you of a previous assault, choose a safe but similar place where you could spend some time. Do your homework to get the most out of your exposure.

For exposures that involve finding a safe but similar place, you will need to distinguish between what *is* safe and what *feels* safe. For someone with a height phobia, for example, sitting on a sturdy balcony or standing near a window in a high-rise building is safe even if it doesn't feel safe. Sitting on the rail around a balcony, on the other hand, isn't safe (and probably doesn't feel safe either). Many people can be honest with themselves about whether something is unsafe or just feels unsafe. If you're having trouble with this distinction, ask a family member, friend, coworker, or therapist to help you decide.

2. Before you begin, practice thought-challenging strategies. Once you have selected and arranged your exposure, practice challenging your anxiety-provoking thoughts before you begin, using the strategies you learned in the last chapter. For someone doing an exposure to traumatic memories of a horrible earthquake, an anxiety-provoking thought might be "If I think about it, I'll lose control of my emotions." For someone doing an exposure involving locking the door only once and not checking it, an anxiety-provoking thought might be "Someone might break in and kill my family, and it would be my fault." Someone doing an exposure to feeling his heart racing might have the thought "I might have a heart attack and die."

When you have identified your anxiety-provoking thought, work through challenging it just as you did in the last chapter, using the Anxiety Thought Record (Form 4.1). Try to prepare your mind with an "alternative thought" that you can remind yourself of during the exposure.

3. Set a specific goal. Those of us with anxiety problems are often our own harshest critics. We sometimes don't give ourselves credit for our successes, focusing instead on what went wrong or what we didn't do. So it's useful to set some goals for the exposure. Then you can look back afterward and see whether you met them.

How can you figure out how to set your goals?

+ They should be realistic but challenging.
+ They should focus on specific actions, not feelings.
+ They should be measurable: someone else should be able to watch and tell you whether you met your goal.
+ The outcome of the goal should be completely under your control.

Here are some examples of helpful goals, as well as some not-so-helpful goals:

Goal	Good or bad	Why
To ask someone out on a date	🙂	This goal is very clear, challenging but realistic, and completely under your control.
To get a date	☹️	While this goal is clear and challenging, it isn't under your control. The person could say "No." He or she could be married, not ready to date, or simply not interested.
Not to feel anxious while making a presentation at work	☹️	This goal focuses on feelings, not actions. It isn't realistic right now to expect that you won't feel anxious. The more often you practice, the less anxious you will feel. Limit your goals to things you do, not things you feel.
To make it through my entire presentation	🙂	This goal is under your control. It is up to you whether to stop. It is an action, and it is something that someone else could measure.

Now that you better understand what kind of goal to set, take a moment to think about your upcoming exposure. What do you feel would be a good, specific, realistic though challenging, action-oriented goal that is completely within your control? Write it down. Remember to focus on actions rather than feelings.

MY GOAL FOR THE EXPOSURE EXERCISE

_____

---

4. Begin the exposure. You've arranged the exposure, identified and challenged your anxious thoughts, and set your goals. Now it's time to actually do the exposure.

Expect some anxiety the first few times (after all, if you weren't anxious you wouldn't be doing this!). Remember to keep the big picture in mind: the small investment you're making now will pay great dividends in the near future.

While you're doing the exposure, pay attention every few moments to how scared or uncomfortable you're feeling. If it's useful, keep track of it on a 0 to 100 or 0 to 10 scale, with higher scores meaning more fear. Don't get discouraged. Though you may notice your anxiety increase initially, or maybe stay the same, if you stick with the exposure for long enough, your level of fear will start to come down. On Figure 5.1 you can see the graph of one person's anxiety ratings during an exposure to riding on a "sea taxi"—a small ferry that takes people across a river or harbor—to confront his fears of being trapped and unable to escape. He was very anxious at first, but, as you can see, as the trip progressed his anxiety level dropped quickly.

Your fear ratings will also drop after the beginning of an exposure, and will usually come down more each time you repeat the same exposure. Remember how that happened for Joseph when he kept jumping off the diving boards?

Finishing Your Exposure and Reviewing Your Goal

Once you have completed the exposure, congratulate yourself! You've begun the hardest, but most powerful, technique for overcoming your anxiety. Facing your fears takes a lot of courage and resilience. You should be proud of yourself.

When you get to the point where you're pleased with your accomplishments, you may want to look back at the exposure. Did you meet the goal you wrote down? Resist the temptation to *qualify* whether or not you met the goal—as in *"Yes, but … "* The anxious mind wants to forget or ignore successes and focus on failures. Here are some

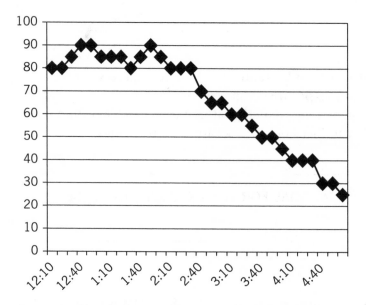

figure 5.1. **Fear ratings during a sea taxi ride.**

examples of qualifications/equivocations followed by statements you can use to challenge such thoughts:

+ "I gave the speech ... but it must have been bad. ..."
  —"I gave the speech!"

+ "I drove on the freeway ... but only because the other drivers stayed clear of me. ..."
  —"I drove on the freeway!"

+ "I stayed in the dentist's chair ... but only because the dentist was being extra nice to me because I seemed so nervous."
  —"I stayed in the dentist's chair!"

Finally, now is a good time to review the anxious thoughts you had before and during the exposure. Compare them to what actually happened. This is important! It will give you extra courage the next time you do this exposure. Use it to remind yourself that while you *expected* something terrible to happen, what *really* happened wasn't nearly as bad as you expected. In fact, most people are often surprised by how well things turned out. Rather than feeling awful and miserable the whole time, it sometimes turns out to be quite enjoyable.

That was exactly Robin's experience when she started doing exposures. Robin had a fear of vomiting, and for years she had not gone out for a meal, either at a restaurant or at a friend's house. She was terrified that the food would not be cooked properly or would be prepared in an unsanitary way, and that she would develop food poisoning and throw up.

Part of Robin's exposure plan was to eat dinner at a nice restaurant with some of her friends. Admittedly, she first checked with the health department to see if the restaurant had received any complaints or poor inspections. The report was clean, but she still felt nervous about going. Robin expected to have a terrible time since she was sure she'd be nervous and on guard during the whole meal. She also expected to get sick, if not from the food, then from worrying so much. With a little encouragement from her best friend, Robin went to the restaurant.

While she felt moderately scared when reading the menu and ordering her meal, Robin soon realized that she was having such a fun time with her friends that she had completely stopped worrying about the possibility of getting sick. Realizing that she didn't get sick and that in fact she had a lot of fun, Robin started trying more and more different exposures and felt full of enthusiasm and courage.

Continuing with Exposure Therapy

If you're wondering what you should do after completing your first exposure, the best thing is to do the same (or a similar) exposure again a few more times. Doing an exposure just once usually won't make an impact on your anxiety. Joseph, the 12-year-old on the diving board, would have remained scared if he had jumped off only once. What got him over his fear was jumping off the diving board many times. Keep practicing over and over until your first exposure doesn't make your anxiety rise above 30 out of 100 or 3 out of 10.

When an exposure no longer makes you particularly anxious, it's time to try something more difficult. There are two ways of proceeding:

1. Just as Joseph moved up to the 5-meter diving board, you could start moving up to the more difficult situations on your Exposure Plan.
2. Start eliminating any actions you take, or things you keep with you, that make you feel safer during the exposures. We call these *false-safety behaviors.* They'll be discussed in the next section.

Here are a few additional guidelines to keep in mind as you plan exposure practices:

+ Exposure works best when practices are carried out *frequently.* In other words, it's better to practice four or five times per week rather than once per week. If exposures are too spread out, each time will be like starting over.

+ Exposure is most effective when practices are *prolonged.* Ideally, your practices should last long enough for your fear to decrease to a mild level, or until you learn that your anxiety-provoking predictions don't come true. Exposure practices typically last between 30 minutes and a few hours.

+ The best exposures are *predictable* (in other words, you know what to expect), as well as under your *control* (as opposed to being forced to confront a feared situation against your will).

Removing False-Safety Behaviors

False-safety behaviors are *behaviors,* or sometimes *objects* or *thoughts,* that we use to control our anxiety when we face situations we fear. They're "false" because they don't actually protect us from any danger; they just make us *feel* safer.

Safety Behaviors and Objects

An example of a false-safety behavior would be the compulsive behaviors that people with obsessive-compulsive disorder (OCD) feel compelled to repeat. These include repeatedly washing their hands for fear that they might have become contaminated, checking and rechecking the doors or appliances for fear that they might not have been locked or turned off properly, or repeating any behavior over and over to get rid of an ominous feeling that something bad might happen.

Though these types of behaviors are among the most dramatic, most people with an anxiety disorder engage in some sort of behavior that they feel keeps them safer. It's not uncommon for people with panic disorder to make sure they keep a water bottle, a cell phone, or a bottle of pills (even an empty pill bottle!) with them at all times. People with agoraphobia often prepare for going out into crowded places by studying maps of buildings or malls so they know where all the exits are. They may take a trusted person out with them to help in case they began to panic. The list of ways in which people try to manage their anxieties and fears is nearly endless.

The problem with these false-safety behaviors is that they wind up actually strengthening the anxiety and getting in the way of your efforts to reduce it. Take a look at the different experiences of Sully and Sally, who both have panic disorder and agoraphobia.

Sully	Sally
Sully has had panic disorder for about 4 years. During this time he also started avoiding public places where he felt he couldn't get help if he started to panic. This includes any number of places, but he lists malls, arenas, and large crowds as his worst situations. Sully began his exposure plan by going to the mall first thing in the morning on a weekday. He figured that the mall would be nearly empty at this time. Sully knew about the need to eliminate false-safety behaviors, but decided that he absolutely needed to keep his benzodiazepine (anti-anxiety) pills with him in case of an emergency. He did leave his water bottle, which he normally took everywhere, at home. "I will do the exposure, but I need my pills as a safety net ... just in case," he thought. Sully went to the mall for about an hour. He was scared about doing the exposure at first, but 20 minutes after he got there his fear started to come down. He figured that if he started to feel panicky or if anything bad happened, he could just pop a pill.	Sally has had panic disorder for about 5 years. Roughly 3 years ago, she found herself avoiding places with large crowds where she felt she couldn't escape if she started to panic. She isn't quite housebound, but she has an extremely hard time going to any stores, malls, or theaters. Sally began her exposure plan by going to some smaller malls at times when she knew there would be fewer people. Sally knew about eliminating false-safety behaviors, so she chose to leave her cell phone at home during the exposure. She also made sure to remove from her purse any pill bottles, as well as anything else that made her feel safe. "I will do the exposure without any safety net," she thought. Sally went to the mall for about 1 hour. Although she felt very anxious at first and wanted to leave, her anxiety came down within 15 minutes. She began to recognize that malls aren't really dangerous places. She became a bit bored with just walking around the mall and found herself going into a few stores.

It might seem that Sully and Sally both had successful exposure sessions. Both went to the mall for an hour, both experienced a decline in their anxiety, and neither had a full panic attack. But what lesson was each learning about the dangerousness of malls? Sally taught herself that the mall isn't a threat. She expected something bad might happen, but it didn't. Sully, on the other hand, taught himself that he can go to the mall if he brings along his medication in case he has a panic attack. Do you notice how that is saying that malls could still be dangerous, especially if Sully doesn't have his medication with him?

Look back at your Self-Assessment from Chapter 2 (Form 2.6 on page 53). What safety behaviors did you list? Since reading more about anxiety, exposure, and safety behaviors, can you add any other safety behaviors to the list? Record your responses on Form 5.5.

Safety Thoughts

In addition to enacting certain behaviors or carrying around safety objects, some anxious individuals also develop safety thoughts or mental rituals that help them feel safer. These may include:

+ Distracting yourself to force the worrisome thoughts out of your mind
+ Repeating phrases, mantras, or prayers over and over in your head
+ Replacing unpleasant thoughts or images with "safe" thoughts or images

Use Form 5.6 to list any safety thoughts you can think of that you use when you're anxious.

Reducing Safety Behaviors and Thoughts

Since this entire book is about helping you feel less anxious, why would we ask you to stop doing things that help you feel less anxious? As we mentioned, safety behaviors may help in the short term, but in the long run they make your anxiety stronger. All the thought-challenging and exposure exercises you are practicing are designed to help your brain *unlearn* that something is dangerous and *relearn* that it is generally safe. Safety behaviors can block that from happening. Take a look at the normal chain of thoughts that happen when people do exposures:

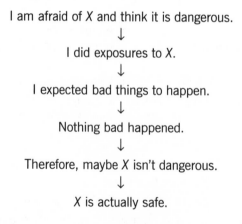

I am afraid of *X* and think it is dangerous.
↓
I did exposures to *X*.
↓
I expected bad things to happen.
↓
Nothing bad happened.
↓
Therefore, maybe *X* isn't dangerous.
↓
X is actually safe.

Now see how safety behaviors interfere with this chain of thoughts:

form 5.5	**My Safety Behaviors**
Anxiety problem	**Safety behaviors**
1.	
2.	
3.	

form 5.6	My Safety Thoughts	
Anxiety problem	**Safety thoughts**	
1.		
2.		
3.		

I am afraid of *X* and think it is dangerous.

↓

I did exposures to *X*, but also used safety behaviors.

↓

I expected bad things to happen.

↓

Nothing bad happened because I used my safety behaviors.

↓

Something bad might have happened if I hadn't used the safety behaviors.

↓

X is still not safe.

What all this means is that as you increase your exposures, you need to decrease (and eventually eliminate) your use of safety behaviors. Many find it best to give them all up at once—this is probably the best idea. Those who find that too difficult should start giving them up piece by piece.

For example, Martha had severe panic disorder and was terribly afraid to go outside her home. She could go out only when she was with her husband. When she started her exposures, she went outside for a walk around the block with her husband beside her. The next time, she went out with her husband trailing 50 yards behind her. The third time, she went around the block while her husband stayed home but talked to her on the cell phone the whole time. The fourth time, he wasn't on the phone but they both had their phones ready in case she needed to call. By the fifth time, Martha went around the block by herself without her phone.

Stopping your safety behaviors all at once is best. Next best is to reduce them as quickly as you can. Safety behaviors will only serve to help your anxiety thrive.

Conclusion

This chapter set the stage for you to begin the most powerful part of treatment: exposure. You learned several important steps:

1. You learned how exposure works and developed an Exposure Plan.
   —The Exposure Plan listed your fears in order from easiest to hardest.
   —You then rated each fear on a 0 to 100 scale to show how much anxiety each item on the list would probably cause you.
2. You learned how to set up an exposure practice:
   —You choose a practice that will be challenging but feasible.
   —You arrange the details of the practice.
   —You challenge your anxious thoughts.
   —You set clear and specific goals that focus on actions rather than feelings.

3. You learned about staying in the exposure until your fear comes down, and repeating the exposure until it doesn't cause any more fear.
4. Finally, you learned about safety behaviors, why they are a problem, and the importance of eliminating them.

The following chapters will give you specific information about how to do different types of exposures. Chapter 6 outlines how to set up exposures to objects and situations. Chapter 7 discusses how to set up exposure to anxiety-provoking thoughts, images, or memories. Finally, Chapter 8 describes how to set up exposures to feared sensations in your body.

6

Confronting Feared Objects and Situations

If your Exposure Plan included facing feared objects or situations (as opposed to feared internal experiences, such as thoughts, feelings, and physical symptoms), this chapter will teach you strategies for overcoming exaggerated fears of virtually anything that is outside your body, including (but certainly not limited to):

- ✦ Heights
- ✦ Snakes
- ✦ Being around people
- ✦ Driving
- ✦ Enclosed places
- ✦ Birds
- ✦ Airplanes
- ✦ Blood or needles
- ✦ Germs

- ✦ Bridges
- ✦ Cats
- ✦ Crowds
- ✦ Forgetting to lock doors
- ✦ Being alone
- ✦ Parties
- ✦ Spiders
- ✦ Open spaces
- ✦ Places where bad things have happened before

- ✦ Certain foods
- ✦ Public speaking
- ✦ Storms
- ✦ Writing in public
- ✦ Darkness
- ✦ Hospitals
- ✦ Messes/disorganization
- ✦ Dogs

Conducting Exposures to Objects and Situations

Exposures to objects or situations are usually easy to arrange, although you may need to be creative. Take the same steps that we described in the previous chapter. After deciding to practice exposures to feared objects or situations (based on your Exposure Plan), you will:

1. Plan the details of how you will find and confront the object or situation.
2. Practice challenging the thoughts you're likely to experience during the exposure.

3. Set specific measurable goals based on actions, not feelings.
4. Start the exposure.
5. Stay in the exposure until your anxiety comes back down.
6. Do not use any safety behaviors or safety thoughts.
7. Finish the exposure.
8. Review your goals and determine whether any of your anxious thoughts or expectations came true.
9. Reward yourself for facing your fears.

The only possibly difficult part of this list is planning out the specific details of finding or arranging the exposure. It can also be tricky to identify variations that might make it easier (for the first exposures) or more difficult (for later exposures). The next section reviews some of the more common feared situations and objects, and provides suggestions and recommendations to help arrange the exposure.

Planning the Details

People can develop fears and phobias related to nearly every imaginable object or situation, including being alone or being around people; enclosed places or open spaces; animal, vegetable, or mineral; and just about anything else on the planet. In many cases, fears are associated with objects or situations that may be dangerous under certain circumstances, yet the fear extends to situations where the risk is small. For example, although driving sometimes leads to accidents, most of the time it's a relatively safe activity.

In other cases, people may fear situations or objects that are virtually never dangerous. We have seen individuals who fear worms, cotton balls, things that are green in color, looking out the window of a tall building, or touching a photo of a spider or other animal. The general process of exposure remains the same regardless of the feared object or situation. Tips for planning exposures for some of the more common fears are presented in the following sections.

Exposures to Places

When a person has a fear of being in or around certain places, exposure practices usually involve going to those places. As you develop your Exposure Plan, it will be important to think of ways to vary the intensity of your exposure to these places so you can gradually increase the difficulty of your practices. If you fear being in a large crowded shopping mall by yourself, you might start by visiting a smaller mall during a slow time, with a family member or friend. Over time, you can work your way up to more difficult exposures by visiting different and larger malls, and by gradually doing more exposures alone (perhaps initially having your "safe person" nearby or available by cell phone).

Table 6.1 gives some suggestions for how you might practice exposure to certain places.

table 6.1. **Practicing Exposure to Places**

Airplanes

Many people have flying fears, but unfortunately exposure to airplanes is becoming increasingly difficult. Safety regulations for airlines and airports limit who can go on or around airplanes without a ticket. Some airlines have special programs to help people with fears of flying, so it might be a good idea to contact airlines to check. Also, some regional airlines offer inexpensive fares for very short flights that you can take advantage of. Finally, there is evidence that computer-administered "virtual reality" (VR) treatments may be helpful for fears of flying. You can find out about practitioners who use VR exposure treatments at *www.virtuallybetter.com.*

Arenas, malls, stadiums, theaters

These types of large crowded buildings are common in most places, although gaining access to them can be difficult without buying a ticket to an event. You may be able to get special permission to enter the building for free during a time when no event is scheduled, or you may be able to practice exposure at an inexpensive or free event. Vary the intensity of the exposure by going to smaller (for example, high school stadiums) or larger (for example, professional or college stadiums) locations. You can also vary the intensity by going during less or more busy times (weekday matinee versus Saturday evening movie) or to less or more popular or busy events (a small symphony performance versus a large rock concert).

Doctor or dentist offices, or hospitals

Depending on your fears, you can vary the intensity of your exposure by going to a small office, a local clinic, a large medical/dental practice, or a major hospital complex. Exposures to medical or dental offices are often fairly easy to set up. Because dentists, doctors, and nurses are health professionals, they may be willing to help you with your exposure practices.

Heights, bridges

Exposure to heights can be fairly easy and safe to plan. Depending on the severity of your fear, initial exposures might involve standing on a stepladder, stool, or chair; on the balcony of a high-rise apartment; or near the window of a tall office building. Some larger buildings, such as the Empire State Building, have public observation decks that you may be able to use for practices. Bridges can be used as well, ranging from small concrete bridges to large steel and cable bridges located over large bodies of water. In some places, particularly mountainous areas, suspension bridges may even be a possibility.

Driving on city streets or highways

There are only a few places left that are not crisscrossed with highways or streets, so finding them is fairly easy. If the amount of traffic is a factor in your fear, start with exposures on less busy roads. For highway exposures, you may want to start with highways that have many on and off ramps so that you can build from staying on the highway for just one exit up to staying on for many exits. As you become more comfortable with smaller roads or deserted highways, you can start moving up toward major freeways or interstate highways.

Exposures to Animals

Animal fears are quite common, but exposures to animals can be difficult to arrange: with the exception of common household pets, most animals live in the wild and may not show up just when we need them! Some animals may be fairly rare in your area, requiring you to visit a zoo or other collection of animals. For some people, playing with fake or toy animals (like a rubber snake) or even looking at pictures or video clips of the feared animal is enough to arouse fear. This is particularly true for people who fear spiders, snakes, and insects.

Please use caution when practicing exposure with animals. If you're confronting your fear of dogs, for example, be sure you know something about the animal (such as using a friend's pet) rather than getting close to a stray dog. Although it's usually safe to touch and hold certain animals with appropriate caution (such as ants, dogs, snakes, harmless spiders), you should avoid handling animals that can cause harm, such as bees and wasps or unfamiliar spiders.

Table 6.2 gives examples of where to find commonly feared animals.

Exposures to People

You can become anxious around others for a variety of reasons. You might be worried about what other people will think of you. You might feel trapped in large crowds. Perhaps a specific person or type of person reminds you of something terrible that happened to you, like an assault or an accident. The advantage of exposures with people is that you can start by asking someone you feel comfortable with to pretend to be someone who makes you anxious. Once you feel comfortable with the role-played situation, you can then practice with someone who normally triggers your fear. Table 6.3 has some examples of how you can plan exposures to feared situations involving other people.

Exposures to Other Objects, Events, or Situations

Virtually any object or situation can become associated with a fear, although some are more common than others. Most exposures to objects and situations are straightforward to arrange, although a few of those listed in Table 6.4 may be more challenging to plan.

Examples of Exposure Plans

Exposure Plans are very individual, so there's no such thing as a typical Exposure Plan. This section provides some examples of other people's Exposure Plans for fears that concern objects or situations. Don't think that your plan needs to look exactly like any of these even if the person described in the example sounds a lot like you.

table 6.2. **Locating Animals for Exposures**

Spiders and insects (for example, bees, wasps, cockroaches, moths)

It may not be uncommon to see spiders and insects outdoors or even in your home, but finding them can be a challenge when you're actually looking for them. Also, if you fear spiders or insects, you may need to ask someone else to catch them for you. Depending on the types of bugs you fear, possible sources include your backyard, garden and plant stores, zoos, university biology departments, beekeepers, exterminators, and natural science museums. You can even order certain specimens through companies that sell biological supplies to schools and researchers (check out *www.carolina.com*). Pictures and videos (check out *YouTube.com*) can be helpful, too.

Cats, dogs, and birds

Often, people with phobias of common household pets, such as dogs, cats, and birds, choose to practice exposure to the pets of their friends and family members. Other sources of these animals include pet stores and local parks or beaches where people walk their dogs, or you might see a bird in the wild. An animal shelter is also a good place to check. They often have kittens, puppies, and adult cats and dogs waiting to be adopted. If you ask, they may let you hold a cat or dog. (Watch out, though: they may try to convince you to adopt the animals!) If you choose to use a friend's cat or dog, you could start with your friend holding the animal while sitting on the other side of the room and then gradually work up to petting and holding the animal yourself. For dogs, you might want to try smaller dogs, such as chihuahuas or pomeranians at first, and then work up to larger breeds like labradors and golden retrievers. It is true that some animals might bite or scratch. Just ask your friends if their pets are ever aggressive.

Approaching or holding unknown animals outdoors is *not* recommended.

Snakes

Finding snakes for exposures can be difficult since they usually hide when people are around. For early exposures, many people find plastic or rubber snakes (like those found in toy stores) to be enough to make them anxious. Most zoos have snake pens for viewing. If you call ahead and explain your situation, the zoo staff may even join you and tell you about the snakes. If you are very lucky, the zoo's professional snake handler may even let you hold a nonpoisonous snake! We have also had success in pet stores that sell snakes. On several occasions, sales clerks have been willing to stay after the store closes (for a reasonable hourly rate) and work with an individual who fears snakes. Because some snakes are poisonous or aggressive, doing exposures by handling wild snakes found in nature is *not* recommended.

Mice and rodents

The best source for mice and rats is often your local pet store. Other possible sources include zoos or the biology or psychology department at your local university.

---

table 6.3. **Planning Exposures with Other People**

Assertiveness

Many people feel anxious when they need to be assertive. Sometimes this means having trouble saying "No" to an unreasonable request. Other times it could involve asking others to change their behavior in some way or to do something for you. Assertiveness can easily be practiced with strangers. Examples include phoning a store and asking the clerk to look up the price of an item, or buying something and then returning it the next day.

Authority figures

Talking to authority figures often feels like a difficult exposure to plan because people frequently think that "bothering" the authority figure could get them into trouble. The fact of the matter is that many people every day talk to people in positions of authority without making trouble. Examples of exposures include calling a police station (obviously, **do not call 911 to practice**) and asking how to file an accident report or register a new bicycle, calling a fire station to ask for directions, and going to a medical clinic and asking the doctor questions.

Crowds

Exposures to crowds are usually similar to exposures involving arenas, malls, stadiums, or theaters. Referring back to that section will be helpful. Other examples of crowded places in which to practice include supermarkets, large restaurants, amusement parks, buses or subways (during rush hour), crowded elevators, flea markets, conventions, trade shows, and busy city streets.

Specific people

It's common to develop fears relating to specific people or types of people after a traumatic event. For example, if a woman is raped, she will very commonly feel fearful around men for a while. If you were mugged or assaulted, it would not be unusual to become anxious or fearful around people who remind you of the attacker. Exposures might begin with interacting with people who remind you a bit of the person or people you fear, and then gradually interacting with people who are more and more like the specific person or people you fear. (*Note*: If someone committed a traumatic offense against you, your Exposure Plan should obviously *not* involve that person. No exposure practices should ever involve doing anything that most people would consider dangerous.)

Speeches

Fear of public speaking is one of the most common fears of all. Fortunately, there are many individuals, groups, and organizations that help people become more comfortable in front of an audience. One of the biggest (and least expensive) is Toastmasters International, which has chapters in many cities and towns around the world (see *www.toastmasters.org*). Groups meet regularly to practice giving speeches. The members can range from people with full-blown social phobia to experienced public figures. For less intense initial exposures, practice in front of a mirror, give a small speech while sitting in front of one or two friends, stand and deliver a speech to a few friends, or even stand up and say a few words at a formal occasion like a wedding.

Sandra: The Need to Check

Sandra often described herself as "a classic OCD case" because she felt trapped by constant worries about cleanliness and would repeatedly check to see whether she had locked the doors or turned off the stove. She estimated that she probably spent about an hour each day going back and checking locks and appliances. She reported showering at least four times and washing her hands roughly 20 times each day. Take a look at Sandra's Exposure Plan in Form 6.1.

table 6.4. **Planning Exposures to Objects and Situations**

Dirt, germs, and contamination

Fears of contamination are very common. Fortunately, exposures to dirt or contamination are easy to set up. This is because for people with contamination fears, virtually everything may *seem* contaminated. Various places that can be used for exposures include kitchen counters, carpets or floors, dusty objects, toilets and bathroom fixtures, objects that have been outdoors, clothes that have not been washed, and so forth. The key to these exposures is to touch or hold the objects and then resist hand washing.

Disorganization and messiness

Fears relating to messes, or having things disorganized or out of order, are often seen in people with obsessive–compulsive disorder (OCD), although anyone can develop similar fears. Exposure to disorganization or messiness involves intentionally rearranging things or making small messes without cleaning them up. For exposures to arouse anxiety, some people need to continue looking at the mess until their anxiety comes down. Others just need to *know* that the mess exists, even if they leave the area. (*Note:* You should discuss this exposure with others living in the same house or apartment before beginning.)

Anxiety concerning locks, light switches, appliance switches, and the like

Most commonly, people develop these fears because they are concerned that they might not have properly locked the door, turned off the lights, or turned off an appliance, and that something dangerous or bad will happen as a result. Exposures usually involve locking the door or flipping the switch once, leaving the area, and resisting the urge to go back to double check that the task was completed properly.

Storms

Of all the possible fears, storms are the one over which we have the least control. It's obviously impossible to ensure that a storm will come along just when you're ready for an exposure practice! Fortunately, weather forecasts are usually accurate enough that you can make sure you're ready for an exposure when a storm comes. When it does occur, make sure you look out the window, step out on your porch, and avoid safety behaviors such as compulsively checking weather forecasts or hiding in the basement. Some people find it helpful to start by listening to sounds of thunderstorms and imagining they're real. In addition, some practitioners may be able to treat storm phobias using VR exposures (for a list of VR practitioners, check out *www.virtuallybetter.com*).

form 6.1	Sandra's Exposure Plan	
Rank order	**Situation, object, or fear trigger**	**Fear rating (0–100)**
1	Touching the toilet and not washing my hands	100
2	Touching a garbage can and not washing my hands	100
3	Touching anything in public places and not washing my hands	99.9
4	Going to bed without checking that the stove is turned off properly	90
5	Going to bed without checking that the doors are locked properly	85
6	Going to work without checking that the stove is turned off properly	80
7	Going to work without checking that the doors are locked properly	75
8	Sitting in someone else's car	70
9	Sitting in someone else's car (a "clean" friend)	50
10	Touching things inside my house and not washing	30

Sunil: Fear of Cats

Sunil's fears were more focused than Sandra's. When he was 11 years old, he went over to a friend's house one evening. His friend's family had a large and beautiful cat that he wanted to play with. When he got near the cat, it turned toward him and the hairs on its back bristled. Then it let out a loud hiss and narrowly missed scratching him. Now, 10 years later, Sunil still gets very anxious whenever he is around a cat.

He has no idea why this event affected him so much. He now lives in an apartment complex and has a neighbor with an outdoor cat. If Sunil sees the cat sleeping near the entrance to his apartment, he feels embarrassed by the fact that he must walk around the building and go in the side entrance. Take a look at his Exposure Plan in Form 6.2.

Miguel: Social Anxieties

You may remember Miguel from the last chapter. He was the man who became very anxious when he needed to talk to people or perform in front of others. Form 6.3 is a reminder of Miguel's Exposure Plan.

Miguel started his exposure with item 10. Calling friends was easy enough to practice, and it was a situation over which he had a lot of control. He decided that he would call three friends every day. He felt that he could call "just to say hi" or he could make up a reason for his call (for example, asking for another friend's phone number).

form 6.2	Sunil's Exposure Plan	
Rank order	**Situation, object, or fear trigger**	**Fear rating (0–100)**
1	Petting a large cat while it is sitting on my lap	80
2	Petting a cat that is on the ground	75
3	Being in the same room with a cat (not petting it)	60
4	Going to a friend's house with a cat in the room	50
5	Walking past my neighbor's cat	50
6	Going to a friend's house with a cat in another room	40
7	Walking into my apartment building if I don't see my neighbor's cat (it might be hiding)	40
8	Seeing cats on TV	30

form 6.3	Miguel's Exposure Plan	
Rank order	**Situation, object, or fear trigger**	**Fear rating (0–100)**
1	Giving a speech at work to the managers	100
2	Performance reviews at work with my supervisor	95
3	Practicing speeches with friends	90
4	Meetings with my supervisor at work	80
5	Playing softball on the company team	70
6	Playing softball on a city league team	60
7	Small talk at work with bosses or supervisors	55
8	Small talk with coworkers	50
9	Calling work clients on the telephone	40
10	Calling friends on the telephone	30

Miguel had a fear rating of 50 (he had predicted it would be only 30) before the first call on the first day, but his fear went down quickly. On the second and third days, his fear about calling friends never went above 15. Miguel decided it was time to start a more challenging exposure. He moved up to calling three work clients every day, rather than getting his assistant to call for him as he usually did, and would make small talk with at least one coworker every day.

Calling work clients was more difficult than calling friends, and his fear rating started around 60, even though he expected it would be a 50 on his Exposure Plan. After five days of this exposure (excluding the weekend), his anxiety rating never got above 30 when calling anyone on the telephone. Small talk with coworkers was also difficult to get going. Miguel realized that he wasn't just nervous about what his coworkers would be thinking about him, but he was also worried that other people would see him talking at work and think he was being lazy. So he modified his plan, and decided to make small talk with a coworker during the lunch break or after 5:00 P.M., when he wouldn't be expected to be working.

The following week he struck up a conversation with a coworker, Rodney, about the local baseball team. Miguel thought the conversation went well even though he could tell that Rodney wasn't a big baseball fan. His fear rating went up to 70 when he started, and came down to a 40 by the time the conversation was over.

The next day, Miguel ran into Rodney during lunch, and started up some small talk about the weather. This conversation went much more smoothly, and they both laughed about all the rain they had been getting. Another coworker, Jill, overheard the conversation and joined in, which Miguel took as a sign that the conversation was going well. His fear rating only went up to 60 this time and came down quickly to 25, although it briefly went back up to 50 when Jill joined the conversation.

Over the next 2 weeks, Miguel started including bosses and supervisors in his small talk, and also started occasionally making small talk during regular business hours. He had noticed that other coworkers chatted briefly at their desks or in the hall all the time, so he figured he wouldn't get in trouble if he did too. He also found a recreational baseball league that he could join as a "free agent," meaning that teams looking for extra players could call him up. When posting his information on the free-agent board, he mentioned that his schedule was busy and that he could probably play only once a week—he didn't want to overwhelm himself with having to go out and play baseball three or four times a week at first. A team called him a few days later, and Miguel agreed to play on Thursday.

Although he felt quite anxious when Thursday arrived, he was comforted by the knowledge that his previous exposures had been successful. He worked on countering his anxious thoughts by asking himself "What is really the worst that could happen? This team won't call me back to play next week . . . and I could live with that." When the game was over, Miguel was disappointed with his performance—he thought he could have played much better—but to his surprise everyone on the team kept asking if he would play again the following week. After a few weeks on the team, he even asked a few of his teammates to go out for dinner after the game.

Bolstered by his success with casual conversations and playing baseball, Miguel pushed toward the top of his Exposure Plan. If he could overcome the easier fears, he figured he could also overcome the more difficult ones, and was thrilled to think that he would no longer be under the control of his anxiety. He scheduled a performance review with his boss and at that meeting asked if he could present the company's quarterly report to the managers. To help prepare, he asked a few friends and coworkers to listen to him practice giving the report. He felt nervous during the practice, but his friends and coworkers all gave him positive feedback. He felt nervous when he presented the report for real too, but when it was finished and he was leaving the boardroom, one of the managers whispered "nice job" as Miguel walked by.

Since that time, Miguel has taken every opportunity to speak up at work meetings. He still feels a little anxious at times, but he now recognizes that almost everyone feels some nervousness with public speaking. It's well worth it to him because he knows that he can beat his anxiety and live his life the way he wants.

Troubleshooting

Of course, not everyone's Exposure Plan will go as smoothly as Miguel's did, although many do when an individual really makes a commitment to the plan. But sometimes an exposure may go in the wrong direction. Even the best public speakers mess up a speech at times (just watch politicians on TV!). Even the cleanest people get sick from a bug every now and then. A dog might bark at you. You might feel woozy when standing near the window in a tall building. In fact, it's best to *expect* that setbacks will happen once in a while during the process. Then you can prepare for them to make sure they don't derail your motivation.

Remember that the anxious mind can play tricks on itself. As discussed in Chapter 4, we often pay attention to things and remember information in a biased fashion. The anxious mind is incredibly good at remembering when things go wrong, but it forgets the dozens or hundreds of times when things go right. Be sure to remember the times when nothing bad happened! It's a useful way of ensuring that you evaluate the actual risk in situations as realistically as possible.

Don't just remember the one time you drove on the freeway and another driver cut you off; also remember the 20 times you drove on the freeway last month when absolutely nothing bad happened. Keep the situation in perspective. Remind yourself that "I only got cut off once in 20 times, and it was just a 'close call.' I didn't get into an accident, I didn't lose control of my car, and I certainly didn't die in a fiery crash like I expected." Then get back on board with your Exposure Plan. Prove to yourself that the negative event was just a fluke or a coincidence.

7

Confronting Scary Thoughts, Memories, Images, and Urges

This chapter provides help when you can't stop intrusive thoughts, worries, images, urges, or memories from triggering strong feelings of fear. Some common examples of frightening thoughts include:

+ Memories of traumatic experiences that repeatedly jump back into your mind
+ Repeated and unrealistic worries
+ Flashbacks to a combat experience
+ Strange or disturbing urges that keep coming to mind
+ Recurring feelings that something bad might happen

Having thoughts like these doesn't automatically mean you have a problem and need to start exposure therapy—everyone has thoughts like these from time to time. But if these types of thoughts *repeatedly* come into your mind, despite your best efforts not to think about them, and if they are frightening to you, then the exercises in this chapter may be useful.

Examples of Common Feared Thoughts, Memories, Images, or Urges

Feared thoughts can take the form of (1) memories of past events, (2) thoughts of bad things that might happen in the future, and (3) thoughts about something happening right now.

Memories of the Past

Having recurring painful memories of past events is extremely common in posttraumatic stress disorder (PTSD). Some examples include:

- ✦ Feeling like your car accident is happening again and again
- ✦ Repeated nightmares about the time you were assaulted
- ✦ Disturbing mental images from the 9/11 attacks, Hurricane Katrina, or some other public catastrophe that won't go away
- ✦ Recurring frightening memories about your time in combat in Vietnam or the Middle East

People without full PTSD can also have recurring upsetting memories even if the memories aren't of an event when their lives were really in danger. For example, people with social fears might have repeated memories about the one time they really messed up presenting a book report in class. A person with panic attacks might not be able to shake the memory of his first panic attack, when he was in a large supermarket and was sure he was dying of a heart attack.

Fears of the Future

Fears of the future usually take the form of "What if … ?" worries. Some common recurring worries include:

- ✦ "What if my spouse was in an accident on the way to work?"—even if there's no reason to suspect that happened.
- ✦ "What if I run out of money?"—even though you have plenty of money in your bank accounts.
- ✦ "What if I don't pass my college classes?"—even though you have received straight A's in all your classes.
- ✦ "What if there's something medically wrong with me?"—even though your doctor keeps telling you that you're healthy.

These worries are common in generalized anxiety disorder (GAD), although anyone—even people without an anxiety disorder—can be bothered by recurring worries.

Urges and Images in the Present

The third type of bothersome thoughts are those that just come to mind and upset you. They aren't memories of bad things that happened previously, nor are they really worries about something possibly happening in the future. They're just thoughts or urges you don't want to have, but that keep coming into your mind. Examples of these thoughts include:

+ Upsetting sexual urges that go against your personal sexual morals
+ Recurring disturbing images of a religious, sexual, or moral nature that come to mind
+ Urges to scream and tear off your clothes in public, even though you would never do that
+ Impulses to count things in a certain way
+ Disturbing urges to say something inappropriate or to hurt a loved one, even though you wouldn't act on these urges

Conducting Exposure to Thoughts, Memories, Images, and Urges

If you read Chapter 5, you already know what's involved in confronting thoughts, memories, images, and urges. The steps involved here are exactly the same. After you decide, based on your Exposure Plan, that you're going to do exposures to thoughts, memories, images, and urges, you will:

1. Plan the details of how you'll find and confront the thoughts, memories, images, or urges.
2. Practice challenging the thoughts you're likely to experience during the exposure.
3. Set specific measurable goals based on actions, not feelings.
4. Start the exposure.
5. Stay in the exposure until your anxiety decreases or you learn that your feared consequences don't occur.
6. Refrain from using any safety behaviors or safety thoughts.
7. Finish the exposure.
8. Review your goals and assess whether any of your anxious thoughts or expectations came true.
9. Reward yourself for facing your fears.

Instead of your usual habit of trying to avoid, suppress, or distract yourself from your scary thoughts, exposure involves intentionally thinking these thoughts. You need to force yourself to think about these thoughts, just as Joseph needed to force himself to repeatedly jump off the diving board in Chapter 5. With repeated exposure, your memories, thoughts, images, and urges will become less frightening and eventually less frequent.

Trying Not to Think about Something versus Not Thinking about It

Try this little exercise. This is Spotty the Polar Bear. Spotty is normally a mild-mannered bear, but he gets *very* upset when people start thinking about him. You don't want to upset a polar bear, so cover the page and do whatever you can not to think about Spotty

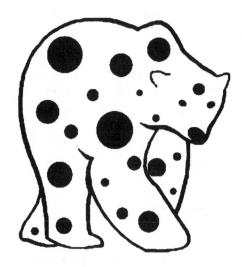

for 1 minute. No matter what, make sure that the image of Spotty does not enter your mind.

How did you do with this little exercise? Nearly everyone thinks about Spotty when they're trying not to. So why is it that when you're trying *not* to have a thought, you can't help but have it?

The human brain is a wonderful machine, but it works in strange ways. Unlike our computers, we don't have a "Delete" key that will get rid of things we don't want. Our brains are designed to think about things, in particular about important things. For some reason that scientists haven't quite figured out yet, when we try intentionally to forget or *not* think about something, our brains put the equivalent of a "VERY IMPOR-TANT" sticky note on that thought. And then our brains keep trying to think that "very important" thought!

It works the same way with disturbing thoughts or painful memories. The more we try not to dwell on them, the more likely it is that we will experience these intrusive thoughts or memories. In fact, the best way to ensure that your frightening thoughts or memories lose their "Very Important" label is to intentionally invite those thoughts or memories into your mind until they lose their power to frighten you.

You're not trying to turn bad thoughts into good thoughts or painful memories into happy memories. Rather, you want to get to the point where you can experience those thoughts without all the fear and negative emotions that go along with them. Let the thought become just a thought, rather than a thought that is perceived as dangerous or threatening.

Exposure to Thoughts, Memories, Images, and Urges

For people with fears of external objects or situations, it's a relatively straightforward activity to develop an Exposure Plan and carry out specific exposures. But people with fears of thoughts, memories, urges, and impulses often have a harder time. Two techniques can be very helpful:

1. People with either distressing memories of the past or scary worries about the future find it helpful to develop worry/trauma exposure scripts.
2. People who have disturbing images or bothersome urges usually do better with forced-thought exposure practices.

We'll take you through the steps of how to develop both of these techniques.

Creating a Worry/Trauma Exposure Script

The goal of exposure to worries or memories is to experience those thoughts repeatedly until they stop carrying so much emotion with them. The exercise with Spotty showed you that trying *not* to think about those thoughts doesn't work. Instead, trying to invoke those thoughts intentionally gradually causes them to lose their power over you, in exactly the same way that a scary movie becomes less frightening if you watch it over and over and over.

Developing a worry/trauma script involves writing out your memory like a summary of a movie, then reading it again and again. Some people choose to record themselves reading the story on a CD or cassette and then listen to it over and over rather than writing it down and reading it. Either way, be sure to include everything that happened (for memories) or everything you fear might happen (for worries)—the full story, from beginning to end. You don't need to do this all in one sitting, but you should devote at least an hour a day to preparing your script until it's complete. The keys to a worry/trauma script are:

+ Write it in the first person:
  —"*I walk down the hall*" instead of "*He walks down the hall.*"
+ Write it in the present tense:
  —"*I walk down the hall*" instead of "*I walked down the hall.*"
+ Write in detailed description with vivid images:
  —"*I can see his angry, pockmarked face as he reaches out and grabs me by the neck*" instead of "*The perpetrator proceeded to grasp me by the neck.*"
+ In addition to images, include all your senses:
  —"*I smell the formaldehyde as I push open the heavy creaking door into the morgue*" instead of "*I walk into the morgue.*"
+ Don't use words that soften the script:
  —"*The officer tells me that they're all dead*" instead of "*The officer tells me that they have all passed away.*"

Most worry/trauma scripts will take several drafts before they're just right and include all the details. You can start with rereading early drafts of your script. But after you've read it several times, add more details according to these guidelines and continue your practices by reading the new version several times.

If you have a lot of different worries, or if you have multiple disturbing memories, briefly describe them in your Exposure Plan form. Rate how much fear (on the 0 to 100 scale) it would cause you to write and read those scripts, and then rank them from 1 (hardest) to 10 (easiest). Then, just like any other exposures, find the point on the Exposure Plan where you feel you can start. As you read the scripts, overcome the fears, and allow the worries or memories to lose their power, you can move up to more distressing worry/trauma scripts.

Pat: Different Worries, Different Scripts

Pat's Exposure Plan for worry scripts is shown in Form 7.1. He decided to list four different common worries and to use two different versions: one that is only moderately detailed (and therefore less frightening) and one that is very detailed (and therefore more frightening).

form 7.1	**Pat's Exposure Plan for Worry Scripts**	
Rank order	**Situation, object, or fear trigger**	**Fear rating (0–100)**
1	Worrying about my girlfriend being killed in a car accident on the way to work (very detailed script)	100
2	Worrying about my parents' health or possible Alzheimer's disease (very detailed script)	90
3	Worrying about my girlfriend being killed in a car accident on the way to work (moderately detailed script)	85
4	Worrying that I don't have enough money to pay the rent and I'll get evicted (very detailed script)	80
5	Worrying that worrying so much will cause me to go crazy and get put in an asylum (very detailed script)	70
6	Worrying about my parents' health or possible Alzheimer's disease (moderately detailed script)	70
7	Worrying that I don't have enough money to pay the rent and I'll get evicted (moderately detailed script)	60
8	Worrying that worrying so much will cause me to go crazy and get put in an asylum (moderately detailed script)	50

People commonly say, "I only have one traumatic memory, and it's the hardest item on my Exposure Plan. How do I find an easier memory to start with?" In this case, it's useful to develop several scripts of varying difficulty by making each draft increasingly more detailed and graphic than the one before. Start with a draft that is manageable. After reading it several times, you'll find that it becomes less frightening. Now develop another draft, with more details.

Veronika: The Worst Fear

Now read Veronika's worry script. Veronika's a 34-year-old married woman who worried every day about a number of things, including her health, her finances, and her marriage. Her worries about her marriage were particularly distressing, despite her knowledge that she and her husband had a wonderful relationship. Even so, she couldn't help but worry that suddenly her husband might find her unattractive and leave her.

Veronika wrote the following worry script:

It's 3:00 on a Tuesday afternoon. My day at work seemed long because I couldn't concentrate due to my worries. I've tried to call my husband to check in and see if he is okay, but I keep getting his annoying voicemail message. I'm tired and stressed, so I decide to leave work early to head home and relax. I pull around the corner onto our street, and immediately see Vince's van as well as a red sports car in the driveway. I don't recognize the car, and I start to feel a nauseous feeling in my gut. I park on the street in front of the house and walk slowly up the driveway. As I pass by the red car, I look in and see a woman's stuff on the dashboard . . . a lipstick case and a hair scrunchy. My heart is pounding and I can almost taste my own vomit.

I walk to the front door and slowly, quietly slide my key in the lock. All of the blinds are drawn, so I can't see in the windows. I slowly open the door and immediately smell a faint perfume. It's not mine. I hear my own heart pounding but then I hear the muffled sounds of Vince's and a woman's voice coming from the bedroom. I gingerly walk down the hall toward the bedroom and press my ear against the closed door. I still can't hear what they're saying, but I hear the woman's voice giggling. I open the door a crack and peer in. Oh, my God. It's what I feared most. Vince is in bed with another woman. And she is so beautiful, not like me. As the salty tears stream down my face, I realize how unattractive I am. She's the type of beautiful woman that Vince deserves.

They both look up, hearing my pathetic sobs. And Vince doesn't even try to make excuses. Why should he? They both start laughing at me as I turn and run out of the house. I keep running down the street, ignoring my car, and find a bench in the park. I sit there alone, crying. And I stay there. Alone, unloved, and unattractive. Forever.

This chilling event never happened to Veronika. But anytime she thought about her husband, this worry would start playing in her head. She would try to snuff it out by phoning her husband (always under the pretense of "seeing how your day is going"), checking the credit card bills for unusual expenses, or doing other things to try to assure herself that it wasn't happening. But the more she tried to get rid of this worry, the more it would come back.

Veronika understood that these thoughts were simply a product of her own mind, so she wrote this worry script and read it to herself twice a day, every day, for a week. The first time she read it, she was an emotional wreck. Her fear rating hit 100 and she couldn't even get herself to finish it. Knowing the importance of doing her exposure repeatedly, though, she pulled the script out again later that day. This time it sent her fear rating up to 90, but she was able to read it all the way through.

The next day, the script was still very hard to face (fear rating up to 75), but she started to notice something. She realized that she had never allowed her mind to go all the way through the worry to the point where she ends up alone forever. She always tried to shut it down by calling her husband to check on him. She thought to herself how absurd it was to think that, even if this happened, she would be alone and unloved forever. The second reading of the script that day caused only moderate discomfort (fear rating: 50), and she started to discover other problems with her expectations. Most important, she realized that the "other woman" in her worries was always an incredibly beautiful woman, like a movie star. Was this the comparison she was using to decide that she was unattractive?

Over the next several days, Veronika kept reading the script two or three times per day, including the times when she started to feel herself begin to worry about Vince. Each time, the story lost some of its power. She remarked that it was like "watching the same scene from a bad soap opera over and over again." And as she kept reading it, she kept recognizing that it was just a story, not reality. Just because she has that thought doesn't mean that Vince finds her unattractive. Nor does it mean that she *is* unattractive. And it doesn't mean that she's going to be alone and unloved forever. It's just a thought.

After a couple of weeks, Veronika was astonished to discover that the script caused barely any anxiety when she read it. She also found that she was better able to let the thought come and go when she started to worry. As she stopped fighting it, it stopped popping back into her mind. And as she became less bothered by the thought, she was able to stop calling her husband all the time to check up on him.

Bill: Flashbacks of Terror

Bill had a different problem. He had served in the army overseas during the Korean War and had had some terrible experiences, including seeing one of his closest friends get killed right beside him. He had carried that memory with him ever since, but never talked to anyone about it. It was simply too hard even to think about. He tried to bury it away in the deepest corners of his mind. For a while he drank a lot and smoked marijuana almost daily to numb the pain.

But Bill couldn't bury the memory. Every time he heard a car backfire, it sounded to him like the bomb that killed his buddy. Every time he heard a helicopter, it took him back to that horrible day. He even had flashbacks when he saw a person of Asian descent because it reminded him of the war.

When Bill finally got into treatment for PTSD, he knew he had to face his demons.

Very reluctantly, he began to write about what happened. His trauma script is very affecting and detailed, so be prepared. Here's a small excerpt:

It is 14:00 hours. Mike and I are on recon, scouting out a possible enemy convoy. Even though we're deep in the bushes, the [expletive] sun is pounding down on us. We're hot, soaked in sweat, and smelling like [expletive]. With all this equipment, M16s, and ammunition I am able to reach down and I pull out my binoculars and look up ahead. It's them. A small unit. They are stopped on the side of the road, but I can't see why. There's probably 10 of them, all heavily armed, standing beside two transports.

I signal to Mike to pull back so we can report in to the sergeant. But then my walkie-talkie squelches. Oh [expletive], I think they heard us. We both drop to the ground motionless, poised to protect ourselves. My heart is pounding and I'm trying to hold my breath so they won't hear me. Seconds feel like hours, just waiting for something to happen. Then all hell breaks loose. The bushes are torn apart by crackling bullets. Wood and mud from the bullets hitting the trees and ground fly all around. We're going to die. A thousand miles from home. Then it goes quiet. Should we run? Stay? What do we do?

Mike and I stay down. There's too much mess around to see if they bugged out or if they are still there. I look over at Mike to see if he can see anything. He is now 10 feet away from me behind a log. He's trying to peek over the log to survey the enemy.

And then he explodes. The [expletive] bastards threw a grenade. The flash is blinding, and the heat sears my skin. I almost pass out from the shock, but I realize I'm covered in blood. It isn't mine. Mike's blood is in my eyes, nose, and mouth. His arm is laying beside me. That's all that remains of Mike. I turn and run. Faster than I have ever run. I don't know where I am going, but I just have to get out of there. Anywhere else but there. I can't tell how long I am running, but I eventually collapse under my own exhaustion in a ravine. I am too tired to move, so I just wait. Covered in Mike's blood. The blood of my best friend. Who I killed because of my radio. Whose body I left out there to rot in this [expletive] wasteland. And now I wait alone, secretly hoping that they will kill me too.

As painful as it was for him, Bill came a long way in his treatment after reading his script over and over. He was finally able to face his memories of that day. They were still horrible memories, but he learned to accept what had happened and allow it to be part of his past. The nightmares eventually began to subside. He began talking to other veterans about their experiences, and found great relief in finally being unburdened of this huge weight.

He was even able to start doing exposures to other things that triggered his memories: he'd spend time near a local heliport, watch movies that showed combat, and eventually even went to a museum exhibit about the Korean War. He knew that he would always be affected by his time in combat, but felt that he was finally able to put Mike to rest.

Creating Forced-Thought Exposures

While some people have memory or worry stories that repeatedly play out in their heads, others just have images or impulses that jump into consciousness. They wouldn't have a story to write out, just a picture or an urge. They can use what we call "forced-thought exposures."

As the name implies, with this technique you force yourself to have the very thoughts you've been trying not to have. By now you have learned that this kind of counterintuitive act can be amazingly successful because of the way our brains work:

1. If we try to ignore or avoid thoughts, our brain assumes they must be very important thoughts, so it keeps reminding us of them.
2. If, on the other hand, we think about thoughts over and over, our brains become bored with them, just as you become bored if you watch the same episode of a TV show over and over.

You're not trying to turn the nasty thought into a good thought, or an urge to do something terrible into an acceptable thing to do, or a horrific image into a pleasant image. The goal of forced-thought exposures is to allow the thought simply to be a thought—a ho-hum, run-of-the-mill thought like any other that might drift through your head without causing you to feel extreme anxiety.

When creating your forced-thought Exposure Plan, there are several questions to think about:

+ "Do I have many different images or urges that I need to confront or just one?"
+ "Are there any situations in which I have that thought and then feel either better or worse?"
+ "If my scary thoughts are about other people, are the thoughts about any particular person more upsetting than my thoughts about others?"
+ "Are there any other factors that might make some exposures easier or harder than others?"

As with all exposures, one of the most important parts is to break it down into manageable chunks and start with the easier parts first. That's what Wendy did.

Wendy and the Image of Her Brother

Wendy keeps seeing horrific images of her brother, Steve, as a dead, mutilated body lying on the ground. As much as she hates these images, she also fears that they imply that she secretly wants her brother dead or even wants to kill him. In fact, she moved out of her family's home and into an apartment because she was scared that she might lose control and harm Steve. She thinks she's an awful person for having these thoughts, and she tries to force the images out of her mind by thinking of other things. That never worked, so she drew up an Exposure Plan (see Form 7.2).

To start her Exposure Plan, Wendy decided that she would intentionally picture the image of her brother's body while she was in her apartment and her brother was at home with their parents. That way, she felt that (1) she couldn't accidentally lose control and hurt him, and (2) her parents would be around in case he somehow did get hurt.

form 7.2	Wendy's Exposure Plan	
Rank order	**Situation, object, or fear trigger**	**Fear rating (0–100)**
1	Picturing the "image" when I'm with my brother and something is nearby that could be used as a weapon (for example, a kitchen knife)	100
2	Picturing the "image" when I'm alone with my brother (no weapon)	95
3	Picturing the "image" when I'm with my brother, but our parents are also around	90
4	Picturing the "image" at a time when I know my brother isn't at home	85
5	Picturing the "image" at a time when my brother is at home alone	70
6	Picturing the "image" at a time when my brother is at home and with my parents	60

She decided that she would picture the image for 20 minutes twice a day. She also remembered about false-safety behaviors (Chapter 5), and decided that she would not call Steve afterward to see if he was okay. After the first 20-minute exposure, Wendy's fear rating was around 90 and she really wanted to call to check on her brother. Fortunately, she resisted checking, and after about 45 minutes her anxiety had come back down to normal.

The second time she did the exposure that day the image didn't cause her as much trouble. Her fear rating only went up to 60, and it came back down to normal within 20 minutes. She did experience some anxiety before going to sleep because she really wanted to call Steve to hear his voice. But she knew she shouldn't. Wendy practiced that exposure twice a day all week, and by the end of the week the image didn't bother her much because she knew that her brother was safe at home with their parents.

Wendy continued to practice the items on her Exposure Plan, gradually working her way up to the more difficult ones. She pictured the image when she knew her brother was home alone for a week, and then pictured it when she knew he was outside. These exposures were hard to do at first, but by the end of the week her fear ratings had always gone back down. Wendy still felt scared about being with her brother while experiencing the thought, worried that she might hurt him. But she no longer feared that just having the thought might somehow cause him to be harmed. To her surprise, she also realized that, other than the times when she was doing her exposure practices, the picture wasn't popping into her mind very often anymore!

Because Wendy and Steve were very close, she told him about these thoughts. Her brother didn't seem upset by them and, after teasing her a little, gladly agreed to help her out with the remaining exposures. They made a plan: Wendy would come over in the evening on days when their parents would be home and force herself to imagine the picture while in the room with Steve. Although this exposure upset Wendy the first time, with her fear rating going up to 100, the second time was much easier.

It became clear to her that there was no way she would lose control and turn into the "fratricidal maniac" she feared. Realizing this, Wendy and Steve conducted a series of exposures in which Wendy brought on the feared image when they were alone together with several kitchen knives in the room. None of the remaining exposures set off Wendy's anxiety.

Now, a year later, Wendy almost never has that image pop into her head. And the rare times when she does think about it, the picture doesn't upset her because she knows it's just a "stupid thought." She sometimes even plays with the mental picture. She imagines the corpse getting up and dancing the cha-cha-cha as a way of reminding herself that it is a silly, meaningless image.

Troubleshooting

Exposures to thoughts, memories, images, and urges can be a wonderfully effective tool in your attempts to overcome your anxiety, but they do present a challenge. The nature of the exercise means that you must confront some very distressing thoughts, and breaking the entrenched habit of having frightening thoughts is no easy task. Changing your way of thinking is one big stride toward success: remember that a frightening thought doesn't mean something bad is going to happen. Nor does a traumatic memory mean that you're about to experience a trauma again. And frightening thoughts or urges don't mean that you are a bad person! A thought is just a thought.

Some people even use a phrase like that as a kind of mantra in their quest to free themselves of their anxious thoughts, reminding themselves again and again: *A thought is just a thought.* It helps them cope with the distress they feel when doing forced-thought exposures or exposure to worry/trauma scripts.

Finally, if you find yourself having trouble doing these exposures, don't get discouraged. Scale back and start with a thought or memory that's a little easier to manage, then keep moving forward bit by bit. You'll be surprised at how much easier it gets. As a friend once said, "Doing exposures repeatedly is therapy; doing exposure once is torture." Each time you practice the exposure, it will cause you less distress and give you more benefit. Trust us: the improvements you make will be well worth your efforts.

8

Confronting Frightening Feelings and Sensations

Almost everyone experiences intense physical symptoms when they are frightened. This chapter is for that smaller group of people who are frightened by the sensations themselves. You should read this chapter closely if your Exposure Plan included facing bodily sensations that cause you anxiety. These could involve a fear of any number of feelings or sensations, including:

- Feeling your heart racing or pounding
- Feeling short of breath
- Blushing
- Headache or other pains
- Numbness or tingling sensations
- Nausea or upset stomach
- Dizziness or lightheaded feelings
- Feeling "shaky" or trembling
- Hot flashes or chills
- Feeling weak-kneed
- Sweating

Different people may fear the same feelings for completely different reasons. Take feelings of sweatiness, for example. An individual with panic disorder might fear sweating as a sign of impending panic attack. Another person with health anxiety might fear it because it's a symptom of malaria. Someone with social fears might fear it because other people might see it as a sign that he or she is nervous. People with obsessive-compulsive contamination concerns might fear sweating because it makes them feel slimy and gross. No matter the cause, if such feelings activate your anxiety, once again avoiding them is not the answer.

The Effects of Avoiding Frightening Sensations

You may be asking yourself, "If I don't like that sensation and I can avoid it, why shouldn't I?" This is one of the most common concerns raised by people who have fears related to bodily sensations. If having a racing heart scares you and makes you think you're having a heart attack, why should you do anything that makes your heart race? Well, there are three important reasons for not trying to avoid the sensations you fear.

1. The sensations you fear represent normal bodily functions. Our bodies are designed to perform certain tasks and to experience certain feelings that keep us functioning properly every day. Our hearts beat faster when our bodies need blood to circulate more quickly (for example, during exercise, when feeling frightened, or for a number of other reasons). We sweat when our bodies detect that we're starting to overheat. We tremble if we're frightened because our bodies release adrenaline. These are all feelings that are very difficult to control because they are expressions of physical functions. These sensations happen regardless of how hard we try *not* to feel them.

2. Avoiding sensations increases your awareness of them over time. By trying to avoid sensations, we actually make it more likely that we'll feel them at a later time. This process is a lot like what happened in the Spotty Bear exercise described in the previous chapter. When we try to avoid something because it scares us, our brains are designed to lock on to an image of that very thing.

And this makes sense. If you were scared because you thought a cougar was prowling around your neighborhood, your brain would shift into "cougar-detection mode." Every time you heard a rustle in the bushes, your brain would scan and ask, "Is that a cougar?" If you saw something moving out of the corner of your eye, your brain would scan and ask, "Is that a cougar?" Normally this reaction is a good thing. You would be extra likely to spot the cougar if it were actually there. And that might give you the extra warning you need to get away from it safely.

But what about sensations that our bodies produce when they're not on high alert? Most of the time we don't notice these run-of-the-mill sensations. If you're sitting down right now, take a moment to notice the feelings of your rear on the chair. Feel your back press against the back of the seat. Before you started thinking about those feelings, you probably didn't even notice them. But does that mean those feelings weren't there before? No, you just weren't paying attention to them.

The fact is that our bodies produce hundreds of different sensations every second. There's the little gurgle in your stomach as you digest food, the beating of your heart, the feeling of air entering and leaving your lungs, the pressure of your shoes on your feet, an itch on your cheek, the taste of saliva in your mouth. We rarely notice such sensations, but if they were to scare us, we would scan for them constantly. And because those sensations are normally there, we'd notice them. And that would scare us.

3. Efforts to avoid sensations can trigger them instead. The third, and possibly most important, reason why trying to avoid sensations doesn't work is that by avoiding those sensations, you often conjure them up! Consider Teresa's story.

Teresa and her husband are in their early 40s. Both are healthy eaters with active lifestyles. Unexpectedly, Teresa's husband had a mild heart attack and, although he survived and is doing fine now, the experience terrified Teresa. "If he could have a heart attack despite his healthy lifestyle, I guess I could too," she thought. Since her husband's heart attack, Teresa has been paying close attention to her body for signs.

One evening, while watching TV, she thought she noticed her heart beating faster. "Oh my God, is this a heart attack?" she immediately thought. Obviously this possibility scared Teresa. Remember back to the beginning of this book where you read about how your body shifts into "fight-or-flight" mode when you're frightened? One of the first things your body does when in fight-or-flight mode is to release adrenaline to make your heart beat faster.

For Teresa, a racing heart leads to the thought that she is dying. This thought scares her even more, which increases the intensity of her fight-or-flight response. This might trigger an even faster heartbeat, as well as other sensations, such as shortness of breath or tingling in her fingers and toes. What do you predict Teresa would think if she noticed those sensations? Would those thoughts make her more scared? And if she did get more scared, what would happen to her fight-or-flight feelings?

Right: they'd get even worse! The fact that Teresa is so afraid of her heart beating rapidly is precisely what caused her heart to start beating rapidly in the first place. This loop in which fear causes symptoms and symptoms strengthen fears can produce all kinds of perfectly natural sensations that can become linked to fears. Shortness of breath can set off people with claustrophobia. Shakiness can upset people who fear that others will see them looking nervous. Those so-called butterflies in your stomach can frighten people who fear they might throw up or lose control of their bowels. Feelings of lightheadedness can bother people who are afraid of passing out.

As a final point, what do you think would have happened to Teresa if her heart had started to beat a little bit faster a month *before* her husband's heart attack? Would she even have noticed it? Possibly not. And even if she had, it probably wouldn't have upset her. At that point, she wasn't even considering the possibility of a heart attack. She might have thought her racing heart was prompted by a cup of coffee, walking around quickly, or being excited about something—and none of these thoughts would have scared her. Because she isn't scared of these thoughts, she wouldn't have experienced a fight-or-flight response, and her heart wouldn't have sped up even more.

So, at the risk of giving you an impossible tongue twister, the point is that *fears of feelings can cause the feelings that fuel the fears.*

Exposing Yourself to Frightening Feelings and Sensations

The methods for exposure to objects and situations, and even to thoughts or memories, may seem more obvious than do the methods for exposure to sensations in your body. After all, if you fear heights, you should go to a high place. If you fear harming your brother, think about doing him harm. But if you fear feeling short of breath, how do you make yourself feel that way?

It's easier than you might think. Psychologists and other mental health professionals have developed a number of simple activities that can safely induce a variety of unusual sensations. These activities are called *interoceptive exercises.* "Interoception" refers to the process of feeling sensations inside your body, such as your heart beating or your muscles tightening. Interoceptive exercises are designed to create those different internal feelings.

The steps involved in exposures to bodily sensations are exactly the same as the exposure exercises you learned in Chapter 5. After you decide, based on your Exposure Plan, that you're going to do exposures to bodily sensations, you will:

1. Plan the details of how you will bring on the sensation.
2. Practice challenging the thoughts you're likely to experience during the exposure.
3. Set specific measurable goals based on actions, not feelings.
4. Start the exposure practice.
5. Stay in the exposure until your anxiety decreases.
6. Avoid using any safety behaviors or safety thoughts.
7. Finish the exposure practice.
8. Review your goals and assess whether any of your anxious thoughts or expectations came true.
9. Reward yourself for facing your fears.

Table 8.1 describes some common interoceptive exercises and the sensations most frequently reported during each one. If you're concerned about hurting yourself when doing any of these exercises, review this list with your physician to be sure they're safe for you. If you have any medical problems or physical limitations (for example, high or low blood pressure, asthma, a cold or chest infection, heart disease, migraines, seizure disorders, and so on), talk to your doctor before practicing these exercises. For most other people, these exercises are perfectly safe, though they may trigger uncomfortable feelings.

Try each of these exercises to see which ones might set off your anxiety. Previous research has found that the ones that most consistently bring on feelings of anxiety and fear include breathing through a straw, spinning in a chair, and hyperventilating. Each of these exercises is effective for at least some people, so it's worth trying as many as you can at least once. Use Form 8.1 to rate each exercise in terms of how much fear or distress it produced for you, from 0 (no effect) to 100 (causing an extreme amount of fear). Once you have them all rated, go back and rank them from least difficult to most difficult (12 to 1).

Look back over Form 8.1 and cross out any exercises that didn't cause your anxiety to go over 30. Then find the lowest ranked exercise that remains and make it the first one you practice regularly. Each time, after you have finished the exercise, write down how anxious it made you feel, using the same 0 (none) to 100 (extreme fear) scale. Keep practicing your chosen exercise until it doesn't cause your anxiety to rise over 30. Then you should move up to the next highest ranked exercise and repeat the process.

If you can, practice each exercise twice a day every day. At the very least, practice it once a day. Naturally, improvements will be quicker with more frequent practice. You can also create your own exercises to bring on the feelings you fear. If you're frightened of your legs feeling shaky and "rubbery" when you are anxious, for example, try

table 8.1. **Common Interoceptive Exercises**

Interoceptive exercise	How it works	Strongest sensations usually triggered
Breathe through a straw.	Breathe through a small straw (a small drinking straw or a stir straw for coffee) for 2 minutes. Hold your nose so that you don't "cheat." This exercise produces a sensation that you are not getting enough air into your lungs.	Breathlessness/ smothering sensations Pounding/racing heart Choking
Hold your head between your knees, then lift your head up quickly.	While sitting, bend forward and put your head between your legs. If possible, keep your head lower than your rear. Stay like this for 30 seconds, then sit up quickly. This exercise works by pushing extra blood into your head. When you sit up, your blood pours back into the rest of your body giving a temporary feeling called a "head rush."	Dizziness or faint feelings Breathlessness/ smothering sensations Numbness/tingling in face or extremities
Hold your breath.	Hold your breath for 30 seconds. This exercise works by setting off alarms in your body that are designed to detect changes in the amount of oxygen and carbon dioxide in your system.	Breathlessness/ smothering sensations Pounding/racing heart Dizziness or fainting feelings
Hyperventilate.	Breathe very quickly and very deeply for 1 minute. Pretend you are trying to blow up a balloon very quickly. This exercise works by setting off alarms in your body that are designed to detect changes in the amount of oxygen and carbon dioxide in your system.	Breathlessness/ smothering sensations Dizziness or fainting feelings Pounding/racing heart Numbness/tingling in face or extremities
Run in place.	Run in place for 1 minute, as if you're jogging. If you have home exercise stair-step blocks, you could also stair-step for 1 minute. As does any form of aerobic exercise, this works by increasing your heart and breathing rates.	Pounding/racing heart Breathlessness/ smothering sensations Chest pain/tightness

table 8.1 *(cont.)*

Interoceptive exercise	How it works	Strongest sensations usually triggered
Sit facing a heater.	Sit 2 feet in front of a small space heater for 2 minutes. This works simply by overheating the body. The hot air also makes it feel more difficult to breathe.	Breathlessness/ smothering sensations Sweating Hot flushes/chills
Spin in a chair.	Sitting in a swivel chair, spin around for 1 minute. This exercise works by temporarily confusing your vestibular apparatus, a part of your inner ear that helps control balance.	Dizziness or fainting feelings Pounding/racing heart Breathlessness/ smothering sensations Nausea
Stare at a light and then read.	Stare at a ceiling light for 1 minute. Then immediately try to read a book or magazine. Staring at the light causes your pupils to constrict to adapt to the extra light. It also saturates some of the receptors on the retina with light.	Blurred vision Dizziness or fainting feelings Feeling unreal or in a dream
Stare at a mirror.	Stare at a mirror directly into your own eyes for 2 minutes. Staring at the same spot for a long time can create odd perceptual experiences and a "tunnel vision" effect.	Feeling unreal or in a dream Dizziness or fainting feelings
Stare at a spot on the wall.	Draw a dot about the size of a dime on a piece of paper and stick the paper on the wall. Stare at the dot as intently as you can for 3 minutes. Staring at the same spot for a long time can create odd perceptual experiences and a "tunnel vision" effect.	Feeling unreal or in a dream Dizziness or fainting feelings

(cont.)

table 8.1 (cont.)

Interoceptive exercise	How it works	Strongest sensations usually triggered
Tense your muscles.	Tense up every muscle in your body—your face, shoulders, arms, trunk, legs, and feet—as tight as you can for 1 minute. Holding muscles tense will cause them to shake while the muscles strain to maintain the contractions. Tensing the muscles through your torso also makes it feel more difficult to breathe.	Trembling/shaking Breathlessness/smothering sensations Pounding/racing heart
Use a tongue depressor.	Using a Popsicle stick or a wooden tongue depressor like your doctor uses, press down on the back of your tongue for 30 seconds. This exercise works by stimulating nerves in the back of your throat that are part of your gag reflex.	Choking Breathlessness/smothering sensations Nausea/abdominal distress

completing a serious of squats until your legs feel weak and rubbery. It's easy to find instructions online *if* you need them.

When the Exercises Alone Are Not Enough

For some people, like James, the interoceptive exercises alone are not enough to trigger fear. James had panic attacks for many years, and he particularly feared feeling breathless. James had learned, however, that his panicky feelings would subside quickly if he was either alone or if he could leave the situation to get some time by himself. He felt particularly optimistic about the hyperventilation, straw-breathing, and breath-holding exercises since they were supposed to trigger feelings such as shortness of breath and smothering sensations.

Unfortunately, James found that doing the exercises at home alone wasn't making him anxious. He recognized that he needed to practice these exercises in places where he wasn't alone, especially places from which he couldn't easily escape if he started to feel anxious. So he bought some coffee stir straws and decided to practice straw breathing while in the mall. He started out at less busy times, and eventually worked up to straw breathing for 2 minutes during the busy weekend shopping hours. He later practiced holding his breath since this was an exercise he could do in public without anyone

form 8.1	**Rating the Exercises**		
Interoceptive Exposure Plan			
Interoceptive exercise		**Fear rating (0–100)**	**Rank order (1–12)**
Breathe through a straw.			
Hold head between knees then lift head quickly.			
Hold breath.			
Hyperventilate.			
Run in place.			
Sit facing heater.			
Spin in a chair.			
Stare at light and then read.			
Stare at a mirror.			
Stare at a spot on the wall.			
Tense muscles.			
Use a tongue depressor.			

noticing. He also attended a professional basketball game and climbed the stairs to his seat very rapidly—an inconspicuous alternative to running in place.

Here are some other examples of how you might combine interoceptive exercises with situational exposure practices for various types of fears:

✦ Spin around in a chair for a minute to get dizzy and then look out the window of a high building (fear of being dizzy in high places).
✦ Wear a heavy sweater during a presentation (fear of sweating while speaking in public).
✦ Hyperventilate in a small closet (fear of feeling lightheaded in enclosed places).
✦ Drink hot soup while in the presence of a group of other people (fear of feeling hot and flushed in social situations).

✦ Purposely make your hands shake while filling out a check or lottery ticket at a store (fear of having shaky hands in public).

✦ Wear a scarf or tie while flying in an airplane (fear of tightness in the throat while flying).

Troubleshooting

Like all exposure exercises, exposure to frightening feelings and sensations can be difficult and distressing at first—they *have* to be in order to work. But bear with them because with time they will get easier and easier. Before long you won't even react to the feelings or sensations. Encourage yourself by imagining the time when they will be no more anxiety-provoking than any other sensation your body produces. Make a commitment to your goal and you'll achieve it.

9

Learning to Relax
Relaxation, Meditation,
and Acceptance

If your anxiety leaves you with a lot of muscle tension and stress, you can benefit from the techniques described in this chapter to help get your body back to a more relaxed state. Relaxation-based strategies are often used along with the other techniques described in this book, including thought challenging (Chapter 4) and exposure (Chapters 5 through 8). They're particularly helpful for generalized anxiety disorder (GAD) and day-to-day stress. For panic attacks, phobias, obsessive–compulsive disorder (OCD), and anxiety in social situations, exposure and cognitive strategies are usually more useful. Nevertheless, relaxation may help to take the edge off any kind of anxiety, making it easier to confront the situations you fear.

This chapter also discusses meditation- and acceptance-based strategies, which are becoming increasingly popular for the treatment of anxiety problems, though the research supporting these strategies is still in its early stages. They can be used alongside the cognitive- and exposure-based strategies you've already learned. In fact, these more traditional strategies can be thought of as acceptance-based techniques in that they help you become more accepting of your anxiety symptoms. As we hope we've made clear by now, fighting your feelings of fear and anxiety, and trying to rid yourself of scary thoughts and imagery, only serve to make these symptoms worse.

In this chapter you'll learn about two types of relaxation-based strategies, progressive muscle relaxation and breathing retraining. (Readers interested in a more detailed discussion of relaxation-based approaches to dealing with anxiety should check out the *Relaxation and Stress Reduction Workbook* by Martha Davis et al.) We'll also talk about mindfulness- and acceptance-based strategies for anxiety. (A more detailed review of these strategies can be found in the *Mindfulness and Acceptance Workbook for Anxiety* by John Forsyth and Georg Eifert.) These books are listed in the Appendix.

Progressive Muscle Relaxation

Progressive muscle relaxation (PMR) is a very popular relaxation technique involving a series of exercises in which you first tense a particular muscle group and then relax it. The alternating phases make you aware of how different your muscles feel when they're tense versus when they're relaxed. People who use PMR report that the exercises help alert them to muscle tension early on, before it becomes intense and more difficult to undo.

The series of exercises takes about 15 or 20 minutes initially. At the beginning, PMR involves alternately tensing and relaxing a large number of muscle groups, one at a time. Once you become better at achieving a relaxed state, you can move to a shorter version of PMR that involves tensing and relaxing several muscle groups at once.

What follows is an example of a "relaxation script." Provided to us by psychologist Debra Hope, it was inspired by PMR scripts that have been used for years by clinicians around the world. It says everything a therapist might say when leading an anxiety patient through PMR. Unfortunately, it doesn't work very well if you read the first paragraph yourself and then try to follow it because you'd have to stop relaxing, read the next paragraph, relax, stop and read the next paragraph, and so on—not very relaxing! Instead, people have found a few options that often work:

1. You can ask a friend or family member to read the script aloud while you follow it. The script should be read slowly, in a relaxing tone.
2. You can read the script aloud into a cassette or digital recorder, and then play it back while following it. The advantage of this option is that you can listen to the tape whenever you want (but please don't listen while driving!).
3. Some companies sell professionally produced relaxation CDs that you can order from the Internet. They're usually narrated by speakers with soothing voices.

Regardless of which option you choose, here are a few suggestions to keep in mind:

✦ Complete the Progressive Muscle Relaxation Progress Form (which follows) for each relaxation practice. Before each practice, rate your level of anxiety from 0 (no anxiety) to 100 (worst imaginable anxiety). After the practice, record your anxiety or tension level again, using the same scale. Keep a record of these ratings to follow your progress.

✦ There are a few steps you can take to increase your level of relaxation, especially in the first few practices. Be sure to practice with your eyes closed while sitting in a comfortable chair (a recliner is ideal). Turn off the telephone, dim the lights, and wear comfortable clothing with a loose collar. After a few weeks of practice, you don't have to go to these lengths—after all, the long-term goal is to be able to feel relaxed no matter where you are.

✦ Once you become more comfortable conducting the relaxation exercises while listening to the script, try going through the exercises without listening to it. This will require you to memorize the exercises, though you don't have to do them in exactly the same order as they are in the script. Conducting the exercises without listening to the script will help you to relax on your own, without requiring you to have someone with you or any special equipment to play the instructions.

✦ As you move through the exercises, try to stay focused on your muscles, your breathing, and your state of relaxation. If any other thoughts pop into your mind, just let them go. Don't fight your thoughts or feelings. Be aware of them, and then let them go.

✦ If there are sounds in the room, such as the buzzing of lights or traffic noise in the distance, just let them go as well. Gently bring your attention back to the exercise.

✦ Some people may feel increased anxiety or even panicky feelings early in treatment, especially those who feel anxious when focusing on the feelings in their bodies. With practice, the exercises usually become more relaxing and less likely to trigger discomfort.

If you prefer to use one of the first two options described earlier (having someone else read the relaxation script or taping yourself reading the script), here's a relaxation script that you can use. It's followed by the Progressive Muscle Relaxation Progress Form (Form 9.1).

Progressive Muscle Relaxation—Long Form[1]

Note: Some words are written in (parentheses) below. These are to guide the reader, and should not be read out loud.

Settle yourself back into the chair. Take a couple of deep breaths and look forward to taking some time to relax. Start to allow the chair to support your entire body.

First I would like you to tense up your feet for 10 seconds by curling your toes up as tight as possible. Keep them curled up and notice the tension in the bottom of your feet and across the top of your feet. … Keep them tense. … You might feel your feet start to shake a little. … (After 10 seconds of tension move on to relaxation.) *Now relax your feet. Uncurl your toes and notice the relaxation and warmth spreading around your feet. … Notice the difference between the feelings of tension and the feelings of relaxation. … Wiggle your toes a little to help your feet fully relax. … Notice how comfortable and relaxed your feet feel. …* (After 20 seconds move on to the next step.)

Now I would like you to tense your lower legs by pointing your toes toward your knees for 10 seconds. Feel the stretch in the back of your calves. … Try to keep your feet relaxed and just tense your lower legs. … Feel the pressure and tightness on the front of your calves. … (After 10 seconds of tension move on to relaxation.) *Now relax your calves by straightening your feet. … Notice the difference between the feelings of tension and the feelings of relaxation. … Notice the tension flowing out of your muscles as your feet and*

---

[1]By Debra A. Hope, PhD. Used by permission.

calves become completely relaxed. ... Feel the warm sensation of the relaxation spreading up your lower legs. ... (After 20 seconds move on to the next step.)

Now I would like you to tense your upper legs by pressing your knees together as tightly as you can for 10 seconds. ... Try to keep your lower legs and feet relaxed as you tense your thighs. ... Feel the tension and pressure on the outsides of your legs. ... Notice how uncomfortable the tension feels. ... (After 10 seconds of tension move on to relaxation.) *Now relax your upper legs. ... Notice the immediate relief as your legs fall back naturally against the chair. ... Feel the relaxation spreading throughout your thighs as they start to feel more and more relaxed. ... Pay attention to the relaxation spreading throughout your entire legs as the tension flows away. ... Allow your legs to feel completely relaxed. ...* (After 20 seconds move on to the next step.)

Now I want you to tense your stomach muscles by pulling in your stomach and abdominal muscles as tightly as you can for 10 seconds. ... Try to keep your legs relaxed and remember to keep breathing. ... Notice the pressure across your stomach as the muscles tense up. ... Notice the pressure and tension across your lower back. ... Feel the tightness in your stomach. ... (After 10 seconds of tension move on to relaxation.) *Now relax your stomach and abdomen. ... Experience the warmth and relaxation that immediately come to your stomach and lower back. ... Notice the difference between feeling tense and feeling relaxed. ... Let the feeling of relaxation flow throughout your stomach. ... Enjoy the sensation of being relaxed. ...* (After 20 seconds move on to the next step.)

Now I want you to tense the muscles in your chest by trying to push the front and back part of your chest together for 10 seconds. Don't shrug your shoulders. ... Just tense the muscles across the front and back of your rib cage. ... Keep breathing but keep the muscles as tense as you can. ... (After 10 seconds of tension move on to relaxation.) *Now relax your chest muscles and notice the difference between feeling tense and feeling relaxed. ... Experience the relaxation spreading out from the center of your chest and back to your shoulders. ... Focus all of your attention on the relaxation in your chest. ...* (After 20 seconds move on to the next step.)

Now I want you to tense the muscles in your hands for 10 seconds by making a fist in each hand and holding it as tightly as you can. ... Notice the tension in your fingers and palms. ... Pay attention to how your fingernails press into your palms. ... Keep your hands tense ... tense. ... (After 10 seconds of tension move on to relaxation.) *Now open your hands and let them completely relax. ... Pay attention to the difference between feeling tense and feeling relaxed. ... Enjoy the pleasant feelings of relaxation in your hands as they rest comfortably against the chair. ... Shake your fingers a little to let all of the tension drain away. ...* (After 20 seconds move on to the next step.)

Now I want you to tense both entire arms by bending them at the elbow and holding them as tightly as possible for 10 seconds. ... As you draw your hands up toward your shoulders, notice the pressure and tension throughout your arms. ... Try to keep your hands limp and relaxed, just tensing your arms. ... Your arms may start to shake a little from the tension. ... (After 10 seconds of tension move on to relaxation.) *Let your arms relax and fall back to your sides. ... Experience the pleasant feelings as the tension flows away. ... Notice the difference between feeling tense and feeling relaxed. ... Focus all of your attention on relaxing your entire left and right arms. ... Allow the relaxation to spread throughout your arms. ...* (After 20 seconds move on to the next step.)

Now I want you to tense your shoulder muscles by shrugging your shoulders for 10 seconds. ... Try to make your shoulders touch your ears. ... Notice how uncomfortable it feels in the back of your neck as you tense the muscles as tightly as you can. ... Keep breathing and keep your arms limp as you focus on tensing your shoulder and neck muscles. ... Hold the tension. ... (After 10 seconds of tension move on to relaxation.) *Relax your shoulders and notice the flow of warmth into your shoulders, neck, and upper back. ... Rotate your shoulders a little to work out all of the knots and tension. ... Imagine the tension flowing out of the shoulders as it is replaced by relaxation. ... Enjoy the calm, pleasant feeling of relaxation. ...* (After 20 seconds move on to the next step.)

Now I want you to tense your neck muscles by pressing the back of your neck against the chair for 10 seconds. ... Notice how the tension spreads from the back of your neck to the muscles in the front and your lower jaw. ... Hold it as tightly as you can. ... Pay attention to the pressure of the tension. ... (After 10 seconds of tension move on to relaxation.) *Relax your neck muscles and experience the warmth of the relaxation spreading in your neck. ... Notice the difference between feeling tense and feeling relaxed. ... Let your muscles go and completely unwind. ... Experience the relaxation spreading across your neck and shoulders as you start to feel more and more relaxed. ...* (After 20 seconds move on to the next step.)

Now I want you to tense the muscles in your jaw and lower face by clenching your teeth together and smiling as hard as you can for 10 seconds. ... You may notice your jaw start to quiver a little. ... Feel the pressure on your teeth and jaw as the tension builds up. ... Keep the muscles tense ... tense. ... (After 10 seconds of tension move on to relaxation.) *Relax your jaw and face muscles, opening your mouth slightly for a moment. ... Wiggle your jaw back and forth a little to let all of the tension flow out. ... Experience the relaxation replacing the tension. ... Enjoy the pleasant sensations of relaxation. ... Notice your muscles starting to be more and more relaxed. ...* (After 20 seconds move on to the next step.)

Now I want you to tense your upper face muscles by closing your eyes and pushing your forehead toward the center. ... Keep your jaw relaxed as you try to wrinkle your brows as much as possible. ... Close your eyes as tightly as you comfortably can. ... Notice the tension and uncomfortable feelings in your forehead and around your eyes. ... Focus all of your attention on the feelings in your face. ... (After 10 seconds of tension move on to relaxation.) *Now relax your forehead and let your eyes return to being comfortably shut. ... Notice the immediate sensation of relief as the tension leaves your muscles. ... Experience the warmth and pleasant feelings as your face and body become more completely relaxed. ... Move your eyes around to let every bit of tension escape as the relaxation flows across your forehead and face. ...* (After 20 seconds move on to the next step.)

Now I want you to go back and tense every muscle in your body at once. Curl your toes and at the same time try to point your toes at your knees. Press your knees together and tense your stomach and chest muscles, make a fist and pull your hands up toward your shoulders. Shrug your shoulders, tense your neck, and clench your teeth. Close your eyes and wrinkle your forehead. Hold the tension for a few seconds, then release. ... Notice the difference between tension and relaxation. ... Pay attention as the tension flows out of your body and the relaxation fills every muscle. ... Enjoy the feeling of being more and more completely relaxed. ... As you start to feel completely relaxed, I want you to focus all of your attention on your breathing ... breathe slowly and deeply, in and out. ... Pay attention to the sensation of the air filling your lungs and then flowing gently outward. ... As you breathe in, say to yourself, "In, two, three." As you breathe out, say to yourself, "Relax, two, three." Keep repeating that to yourself. ... In ... two ... three. ... Relax ... two ... three. ...

In ... two ... three. ... Relax ... two ... three. ...
In ... two ... three. ... Relax ... two ... three. ...
In ... two ... three. ... Relax ... two ... three. ...
In ... two ... three. ... Relax ... two ... three. ...

Continue breathing in and out slowly and evenly. Forget about everything else and just concentrate on being relaxed and breathing. ... Keep counting as you breathe in and out. ... Let all of your muscles go and think only of feeling totally and completely relaxed. ... Notice the sensation of the chair pressing against the back of your legs, your hips, your back, and your head. ... Settle back and let the chair completely support you. ... Pay attention to the sensations of relaxation throughout your body. ... Feeling calm, peaceful, and relaxed. ... Now I am going to count from one to five. As I count you will become more completely relaxed. ... One ... feeling comfortable and relaxed ... two ... enjoying those pleasant sensations ... three ... letting every tension leave your body ... four ... feeling more calm ... five ... feeling completely relaxed. ... Continue feeling totally relaxed as you focus all of your concentration on your breathing. ... Keep counting in ... two ... three. ... Relax ... two ... three. ... (Let this go on as you relax and count your breathing for 1 to 2 minutes more.)

Now I am going to count from five to one. When I get to two, open your eyes. As I count backward you will start to feel more alert but still completely relaxed. ... Five ... feeling relaxed and peaceful ... four ... start to become a bit more aware of your surroundings but still remain relaxed ... three ... notice the sounds in the room as you become more alert ... two, open your eyes. Become more and more alert but warm, peaceful, and relaxed. ... One ... relaxed but fully alert.

You should practice PMR regularly to get the most benefit. Learning to relax is a skill, just like learning to play the piano or learning to swim. Don't expect it to work perfectly the first time. Just keep practicing. Most experts recommend practicing once or twice daily. Soon you'll find that you're developing good control over your feelings of anxiety and tension.

After a few weeks of practicing the long form of the script, when you find it easier to become relaxed, try the shorter version. Again, have someone read it to you or record it on a tape or CD. Make sure you continue rating your anxiety/tension before and after you practice relaxing. Once you're comfortable completing the exercises while listening to the instruction, try practicing without listening to it.

form 9.1	**Progressive Muscle Relaxation Progress Form**	

Mark your ratings on a scale from 0 (no anxiety) to 100 (worst imaginable anxiety).

Date/time	Anxiety/tension before	Anxiety/tension after

Progressive Muscle Relaxation—Short Form[2]

Note: Some words are written in (parentheses) below. These are to guide the reader, and should not be read out loud.

Settle yourself back into the chair. Take a couple of deep breaths and look forward to taking some time to relax. Start to allow the chair to support your entire body.

First I would like you to tense up your hands, feet, arms, and legs. Curl your toes and point them toward your knees. Press your knees together. Make fists and bend your elbows. Notice the tension across the top of your feet and the stretch in your calves and thighs. ... Pay attention to your fingers pressing into your palms. ... Keep your arms and legs tense. ... (After 10 seconds of tension move on to relaxation.) *Now relax your arms and legs. Uncurl your toes and stretch out your feet and legs. ... Notice the pleasant feelings of relaxation in your hands and arms as they rest comfortably against the chair.* (After 20 seconds move on to the next step.)

Now I want you to tense your stomach muscles and chest. Hold in your stomach and try to push the front and back walls of your chest together as tightly as you can for 10 seconds. ... Try to keep your legs relaxed and remember to keep breathing. ... Don't shrug your shoulders but notice the pressure across your stomach as the muscles tense up. ... Notice the pressure and tension across your back. ... Feel the tightness. ... (After 10 seconds of tension move on to relaxation.) *Now relax your stomach, abdomen, and chest. ... Experience the warmth and relaxation that immediately come to your stomach and back. ... Notice the difference between feeling tense and feeling relaxed. ... Let the feeling of relaxation flow throughout your chest and stomach. ... Enjoy the sensation of being relaxed. ...* (After 20 seconds move on to the next step.)

Now I want you to tense your shoulder muscles by shrugging your shoulders for 10 seconds. ... Try to make your shoulders touch your ears. ... Notice how uncomfortable it feels in the back of your neck as you tense the muscles as tightly as you can. ... Keep breathing and keep your arms limp as you focus on tensing your shoulder and neck muscles. ... Hold the tension. ... (After 10 seconds of tension move on to relaxation.) *Relax your shoulders and notice the flow of warmth into your shoulders, neck, and upper back. ... Rotate your shoulders a little to work out all of the knots and tension. ... Imagine the tension flowing out of the shoulders as it is replaced by relaxation. ... Enjoy the calm, pleasant feeling of relaxation. ...* (After 20 seconds move on to the next step.)

Now I want you to tense your neck muscles by pressing the back of your neck against the chair and tense the muscles in your jaw and lower face by clenching your teeth together and smiling as hard as you can. Tense the rest of your face by closing your eyes and pushing your forehead toward the center, wrinkling your brow as much as possible. ... Notice how the tension spreads from the back of your neck across your face. ... Hold it as tightly as you can. ... (After 10 seconds of tension move on to relaxation.) *Relax your face and neck muscles and experience the warmth of the relaxation spreading. ... Move your eyes and your jaw back and forth a little to let all of the tension flow out. ... Experience*

_____
[2]By Debra A. Hope, PhD. Used by permission.

the relaxation spreading across your forehead, neck, and shoulders as you start to feel more and more relaxed. ... (After 20 seconds move on to the next step.)

Now I want you to go back and tense every muscle in your body at once. Curl your toes and at the same time try to point your toes at your knees. Press your knees together and tense your stomach and chest muscles, make a fist and pull your hands up toward your shoulders. Shrug your shoulders, tense your neck, and clench your teeth. Close your eyes and wrinkle your forehead. Hold the tension for a few seconds, then release. ... Notice the difference between tension and relaxation. ... Pay attention as the tension flows out of your body and the relaxation fills every muscle. ... Enjoy the feeling of being more and more completely relaxed. ... As you start to feel completely relaxed, I want you to focus all of your attention on your breathing. ... Breathe slowly and deeply, in and out. ... Pay attention to the sensation of the air filling your lungs and then flowing gently outward. ... As you breathe in, say to yourself, "In, two, three." As you breathe out, say to yourself, "Relax, two, three." Keep repeating that to yourself. ... In ... two ... three. ... Relax ... two ... three ...

In ... two ... three. ... Relax ... two ... three ...
In ... two ... three. ... Relax ... two ... three ...
In ... two ... three. ... Relax ... two ... three ...
In ... two ... three. ... Relax ... two ... three ...

Continue breathing in and out slowly and evenly. Forget about everything else and just concentrate on being relaxed and breathing. ... Keep counting as you breathe in and out. ... Let all of your muscles go and think only of feeling totally and completely relaxed. ... Notice the sensation of the chair pressing against the back of your legs, your hips, your back, and your head. ... Settle back and let the chair completely support you. ... Pay attention to the sensations of relaxation throughout your body. ... Feeling calm, peaceful, and relaxed. ... Now I am going to count from one to five. As I count you will become more completely relaxed. ... One ... feeling comfortable and relaxed ... two ... enjoying those pleasant sensations ... three ... letting every tension leave your body ... four ... feeling more calm ... five ... feeling completely relaxed. ... Continue feeling totally relaxed as you focus all of your concentration on your breathing. ... Keep counting in ... two ... three. ... Relax ... two ... three. ... (Let this go on as you relax and count your breathing for 1 to 2 minutes more.)

Now I am going to count from five to one. When I get to two open your eyes. As I count backward you will start to feel more alert but still completely relaxed. ... Five ... feeling relaxed and peaceful ... four ... start to become a bit more aware of your surroundings but still remain relaxed ... three ... notice the sounds in the room as you become more alert ... two, open your eyes. Become more and more alert but warm, peaceful, and relaxed. ... One ... relaxed but fully alert.

Keep practicing the short version until it works as well as the longer one. Then, for a final step, try the full-body form of the exercise. It's brief and easy to use when you don't have a lot of time. Start with a tape or CD recording (or someone reading the instructions). Then practice on your own, without the recording. Begin your practices in a relaxing environment (eyes closed, comfortable chair and clothing, quiet room), and gradually progress to practicing in less relaxing environments.

Progressive Muscle Relaxation—Full-Body Form[3]

Settle yourself back into the chair. Take a couple of deep breaths and look forward to taking some time to relax. Start to allow the chair to support your entire body.

Now I want you to go back and tense every muscle in your body at once. Curl your toes and at the same time try to point your toes at your knees. Press your knees together and tense your stomach and chest muscles, make a fist and pull your hands up toward your shoulders. Shrug your shoulders, tense your neck, and clench your teeth. Close your eyes and wrinkle your forehead. Hold the tension for a few seconds, then release. . . . Notice the difference between tension and relaxation. . . . Pay attention as the tension flows out of your body and the relaxation fills every muscle. . . . Enjoy the feeling of being more and more completely relaxed. . . . As you start to feel completely relaxed, I want you to focus all of your attention on your breathing. . . . Breathe slowly and deeply, in and out. . . . Pay attention to the sensation of the air filling your lungs and then flowing gently outward. . . . As you breathe in, say to yourself, "In, two, three." As you breathe out, say to yourself, "Relax, two, three." Keep repeating that to yourself. . . . In . . . two . . . three. . . . Relax . . . two . . . three. . . .

Breathing Retraining

You may have noticed that when you're under a lot of stress or anxiety, your breathing becomes more rapid and shallow. This can sometimes lead to shortness of breath, a normal component of the fight-or-flight response (discussed in Chapter 1). Unlike other changes that occur during the fight-or-flight response (for example, the release of adrenalin, changes in heart rate, changes in liver activity), breathing is under our own control. In fact, breathing is one of the few systems in the body that is both involuntary (it keeps going even if you aren't thinking about it, such as when you are asleep) and voluntary (you can directly control it, such as by blowing or holding your breath). So when the fight-or-flight response instigates speeded-up breathing through the *involuntary* system, you can regain control of your breath by using a *voluntary* override.

How Does Breathing Work?

A silly question . . . our lungs suck in air and then blow it back out, right? That's how many people think about their breathing—and it's entirely false. We don't actually have any muscles for sucking in air or blowing it back out. Believe it or not, our lungs are essentially glorified grocery bags. Breathing comes from two groups of muscles that don't even touch the lungs. Instead, they expand or shrink our chest "cavity," which

---

[3]By Debra A. Hope, PhD. Used by permission.

is the inside part of our bodies, extending from the shoulders roughly down to the stomach.

These groups of muscles are the *intercostal muscles* and the *diaphragm*. The intercostals are a series of muscles that line the rib cage. The diaphragm is a large muscle that completely separates the upper part of the inside of your body from your abdomen, which houses the stomach, intestines, and so on. The main job of the intercostals is to expand and contract the rib cage. The job of the diaphragm, which is shaped like a dome or an upside-down bowl, is to flatten itself. Why would they do that?

Well, air likes balance. If air had its way, it would exist in the same amount at the same pressure everywhere. But this can't always be the case, so air will rush out of areas of higher pressure into areas with lower pressure in an effort to achieve balance. Think of the terrible time air has when dealing with an accordion. When the accordion is pulled apart, it creates a large space with little air in it. The air rushes in from outside the accordion (making that much-maligned accordion sound) to try to achieve balance. Then, of course, the accordionist pushes the instrument back together, creating a lot less space and more air pressure. The air forces itself out (again, making music).

A similar process occurs with breathing. When we want air to rush into our lungs, our intercostals expand the rib cage and the diaphragm flattens. This creates more space inside the chest cavity. Since air seeks to have a balance in pressure in the lungs and outside the body, air rushes in to fill the lungs. When we exhale, the intercostals and diaphragm return to normal, thereby shrinking the space inside our chests and the air rushes out. When we need to blow hard, the intercostals can actually pull the ribs closer together to force even more air out.

Try it. Put your hands on your ribs just under your armpits. Now blow out until you don't have any air left. Notice how tight and pulled in your ribs feel? Now inhale normally, and feel the ribs expand back out.

What does all this have to do with anxiety or relaxation? A lot, actually. When the fight-or-flight response is turned on, most of our breathing comes from the intercostals, not the diaphragm. This is because our body is trying to saturate itself with oxygen for the muscles, to prepare the body to escape or fight. Fast, shallow breathing gets the oxygen in quickly and forces out a lot of carbon dioxide.

The diaphragmatic breathing exercise describes a "breathing retraining" technique that can help reduce the symptoms caused by overbreathing. It involves breathing slowly, using your diaphragm rather than your intercostal muscles. There is also a meditational component that will help you stay focused on the exercise. Note that there are different approaches to breathing retraining—this is just one variation. You may have already learned a slightly different approach during therapy, yoga classes, singing lessons, or elsewhere.

Diaphragmatic Breathing Exercise

To begin, find a spot where you can lie down comfortably on your back. Now, place your left hand palm-down over your belly button. Take your right hand and place it on your chest. Breathe normally through your nose. Notice how your hands are moving up and down in rhythm with your breathing. If you are relaxed right now, both hands are probably moving up and down as you breathe in and out.

For the first part of the exercise, pretend you are walking around on a crowded beach. This means, of course, that you should suck in your belly and stick out your chest. (Don't worry—everybody does this!) Now breathe while still holding your stomach tight. Notice that only the hand on your chest is moving up and down now? This is essentially what is happening when you get anxious and begin to breathe mostly from your chest. And notice how uncomfortable this feels, and how you don't feel you're getting enough air. Does this cause you any feelings of anxiety or discomfort?

Now, allow your bottom hand to move up and down again as you breathe. Focus on your breathing, inhaling slowly and deeply so that your diaphragm gets involved and your lower hand rises. Notice how much more air you're taking in, and notice the feeling of relaxation and calmness that comes along with it. Notice how different this feels from the chest breathing. Continue breathing slowly, in and out, for 2 minutes.

For the last part of the exercise, you're going to add a component to help you focus on the exercise and increase your relaxation. Each inhalation should take about 4 seconds, as should each exhalation (if 4 seconds seems too short, you can extend the time to 5 or 6 seconds for each inhalation and each exhalation). As you inhale, mentally repeat the word "inhale" followed by the numbers 2, 3, and 4, as you count the number of seconds spent inhaling. As you exhale, mentally repeat the word "relax" followed by the numbers 2, 3, and 4, as you count the number of seconds spent exhaling. Don't hold your breath in between each inhale and exhale. Rather, keep the cycle of inhaling and exhaling smooth and relaxed.

Inhale–2–3–4
Relax–2–3–4
Inhale–2–3–4
Relax–2–3–4
Inhale–2–3–4
Relax–2–3–4

Continue the practice for about 10 minutes and do it at least twice a day.

A word of caution about breathing retraining. Although it can be a useful strategy for dealing with general anxiety, worry, tension, and stress, it should *not* be used as an avoidance strategy. If you're afraid of feeling panicky and breathless, for example, don't tell yourself, "Oh, no ... I'm having a panic attack ... I better slow down my breathing so I don't faint or drop dead!" This just turns breathing retraining into a safety behavior that will help your anxiety to thrive.

If you find that you're doing the breathing exercises out of fear of what might happen if you don't do them, then don't do them! (If this distinction is confusing you, please reread Chapter 5, on exposure.) But it's perfectly appropriate to use them to deal with general anxiety and stress (for example, feeling worried about all your deadlines at work, feeling stressed out by your screaming children, and so on).

Mindfulness- and Acceptance-Based Strategies

The last strategy in this chapter, mindfulness and acceptance, is not so much a technique as way to react to anxious thoughts, worries, or unpleasant emotions. There are lots of different techniques for achieving a state of mindfulness and acceptance, including some of the other strategies described throughout this book.

When we experience negative emotions or anxiety-provoking thoughts, we usually try to get rid of them by mentally pushing them out of our minds. Sadly, though, this rarely works. Trying to force out thoughts or emotions usually only makes them come back stronger than before. (This problem was discussed in detail in Chapter 7.) Mindfulness and acceptance, on the other hand, emphasize the importance of *not fighting* your thoughts and feelings. After all, they are just thoughts and feelings—they're part of who you are, part of what it means to be human.

Think of it this way: Picture a scene where you are looking at a river. Imagine that your thoughts or emotions are a boat floating down the river. But you don't want the boat to block your view of the river. You could try wading into the water and holding back the boat. How effective do you think that would be? You probably would burn up a lot of energy and effort, but the boat would float along anyway. You might even slow it down slightly, which would keep it in your view even longer!

Another approach would be to get behind the boat and try to push it out of your view. Would that work? Again, probably not. You would waste a lot of time and energy without making the boat float away any faster.

Or you could allow yourself to accept that the boat is coming and that it will go away eventually. Rather than fighting the boat or getting angry about it, you could watch it come and watch it leave. You can be aware of the boat, without judging it. Look at the boat. Does it have a motor or sail? How big is the boat? How deep does it sit in the water? Is there anybody on the deck of the boat?

This is the heart of mindfulness and acceptance. You may not want negative emotions or anxious thoughts, but don't fight them. Sit back, let them float along your "mental river," and let them float away. This can feel strange at first because we're so used to trying *not* to have these thoughts or feelings. But with practice, you can become an expert at letting the thoughts and emotions easily come and go. You'll be surprised by how quickly they float away when you don't fight them!

There are a number of strategies for achieving a state of mindfulness and acceptance. Some include employing images and metaphors similar to the boat metaphor; some focus on meditation. You can find some excellent books and CDs if you'd like to learn more about mindfulness-based meditation (see the Appendix for some suggestions). Many of the strategies already described in this book (including exposure and some of the cognitive strategies) can be used to promote a state of acceptance or mindfulness.

For example, decatastrophizing (a cognitive strategy you read about in Chapter 4) helps you accept an upsetting situation or feeling, recognizing that feared outcomes are often not as bad as they seem. Similarly, imaginal exposure (Chapter 7) and interoceptive exposure (Chapter 8) teach us to be aware of and accept our uncomfortable thoughts and feelings, rather than trying to change them. So if you've been practicing these techniques, you've already been involved with mindful acceptance even if you didn't know it.

Conclusion

Relaxation-based strategies often feel great—it's no surprise that they're among the most popular techniques for treating anxiety. But they're *not* a substitute for thought challenging (Chapter 4) and exposure (Chapters 5 through 8). In most cases, those are the keys to overcoming anxiety. Use the relaxation skills described in this chapter to deal with general feelings of anxiety and stress, but do not rely on them exclusively as strategies for coping with more focused fears, panic attacks, OCD symptoms, and the like.

Relaxation is a skill and, like any skill, you won't get good at it unless you practice. Many people don't become completely relaxed after first trying these exercises; some get no benefit at first. Keep practicing, though—it will become easier and easier to slow down your body and mind and have one more tool at your disposal to control your anxiety.

10

Medications and Herbal Remedies

So far we have been emphasizing strategies for reducing anxiety by changing your thoughts and behaviors. There's strong evidence that medications can also lead to significant reductions in anxiety and fear. This chapter will help you decide whether medications are right for you and to understand which medications are most helpful for which forms of anxiety. The chapter also provides a recap of herbal remedies and other alternative or complementary treatments for anxiety.

It's amazing how many people treat medications for anxiety or depression differently from medications for other illnesses, stopping them or changing dosage without consulting their doctors. You can't begin such medications without a doctor's advice, and you shouldn't change or stop them without a doctor's advice. *Any* decisions you make about *any* medications should be done in consultation with your doctor or other prescribing practitioner.

Myths and Misconceptions

Not surprisingly, people who are anxious in general are often reluctant to take medications, including anti-anxiety drugs and antidepressants (both of which are frequently prescribed for anxiety-based problems). Some of that reluctance stems from beliefs that might be untrue. Here are some common myths and misconceptions about medications, as well as information to set the record straight.

Myth: "Medications will make me sick, or worse!"
Reality: Almost any medication comes with possible risks to your health, though the chances of having serious problems in response to taking a medication are very small. The benefits far outweigh the risks, or your doctor would not have prescribed it. Medications approved for anxiety and related problems by government regulatory bodies (for example, the Food and Drug Administration [FDA] in the United States) can't be marketed until they have been extensively tested for both effectiveness and safety.

Even the medications you read about that are later pulled from the market for possible problems usually pose a danger to only a small minority of patients. For example, sale of the antidepressant nefazodone (Serzone) was discontinued in the United States by the manufacturer (Bristol-Myers Squibb) in 2004 owing to the possibility of liver failure, which occurred in 1 in 250,000 to 300,000 patient-years. (A *patient-year* refers to the sum of each patient's exposure expressed in years; for example, two patients taking the drug for 6 months each would equal 1 patient-year.) Although such risks are very slight, it's important to remain under the care of a physician who can determine whether you fall in that small group. And don't forget that side effects of certain medications may mimic the physical symptoms of anxiety, which may lead you to think that your anxiety is worsening. Often these side effects diminish over time.

Myth: "Medications will make me suicidal."

Reality: In recent years, the FDA has issued a "black-box warning" highlighting the risk of suicide with antidepressant use in children, adolescents, and young adults (ages 18–24). In part, this warning was based on a review of 24 studies that found the combined risk of suicidal thoughts to be 4% for young patients taking antidepressants, compared with 2% for those taking placebo. There was no increase in actual suicide attempts or completed suicides. And the increased risk of suicidal thoughts did not appear in adults over 24.

Scientists argue that the benefits of antidepressants far outweigh their risks for those, including children, who need them. For the majority of individuals, antidepressants actually *decrease* the risk of suicide. Keep in mind that most people who attempt suicide are not taking antidepressants, and many people who feel suicidal report feeling less so when taking antidepressants. In fact, countries with higher rates of antidepressant use have been found to have lower suicide rates in children ages 5 to 14.

Myth: "Having to take medications for anxiety means that I'm weak."

Reality: Taking medications for anxiety is no more a sign of weakness than taking medications for high blood pressure or heart disease is weak. And many people truly need them. According to the U.S. Centers for Disease Control and Prevention (CDC), almost 118 million of the 2.4 billion drugs prescribed during visits to doctors and hospitals in 2005 were for antidepressants, making them the most commonly prescribed medications in the United States.

Myth: "I'll be on antidepressants or anti-anxiety medications for the rest of my life."

Reality: A return of anxiety symptoms is more common after stopping medication than after stopping psychological treatments (such as cognitive-behavioral therapy [CBT]), true, but many people are able to decrease their dosage or discontinue their medications entirely without relapsing, particularly if they reduce their dosage gradually under a doctor's guidance.

Myth: "Taking such medications will change my personality."

Reality: Most people who take medications for anxiety report that they still feel like themselves. Some even say that it was their anxiety that had changed their personalities, and the medication made them feel more like their old selves.

Myth: "The side effects will be unbearable."
Reality: Looking at the long list of possible side effects associated with just about any medication is scary. In reality, though, (1) most people experience only a small number of side effects, if any; (2) the severity of the side effects is usually manageable; (3) many side effects tend to improve over time—those that don't can often be managed by lowering the dosage; and (4) if side effects are intolerable, you can work with your doctor to switch to a different medication or taper off completely.

Myth: "I will become addicted."
Reality: Some medications can make you uncomfortable when you discontinue them, especially if you stop them abruptly. This is not necessarily addiction, but it can make it hard to stop. Most people do succeed in going off them, especially if they reduce the dosage gradually under medical supervision.

Note that antidepressant medications (the most commonly prescribed drugs for treating anxiety problems) are *not* associated with "tolerance"—the need to keep increasing the dose to achieve the same benefit—which is one of the hallmarks of an addictive drug.

Advantages and Disadvantages of Medication Treatments

Among the potential benefits of taking medication for anxiety:

✦ Research on the treatment of anxiety-based problems has consistently found that medication treatments reduce their severity, in some cases eliminating the problem completely.

✦ Medications are relatively easy to get: any physician, not just a psychiatrist, can prescribe them. In contrast, it can sometimes be difficult to find a qualified cognitive-behavioral therapist.

✦ Medications work relatively quickly: anti-anxiety medications typically work within minutes or hours, and antidepressants usually start working within a few weeks. CBT can take weeks or months to have an effect.

✦ Medications are often less expensive than CBT, at least over the short term (in the long term, CBT is often less expensive).

✦ Taking medications does not require much effort. All you have to do is remember to take a pill. In contrast, CBT requires hours of therapy, as well as completion of daily homework assignments.

Now, what's the downside of taking medication?

✦ Medication treatments do not work well for every type of anxiety problem. For example, they don't appear to be successful with specific phobias (fears of animals, blood, needles, or heights). And even for anxiety problems that generally respond well, the medication won't work for everyone.

+ Relapse rates are higher after stopping medication than they are after stopping CBT. In other words, although CBT and medications work about equally well in the short term, CBT often has better staying power once treatment has stopped.

+ People typically continue to take their medications for a much longer period than they usually remain in CBT. Therefore, over the long term, the costs of medication treatment are often higher than the costs of CBT.

+ Medication treatments are often associated with uncomfortable side effects, particularly at higher doses (though, to be fair, CBT can also have "side effects" early in treatment, including feelings of anxiety, nightmares, irritability, and fatigue).

+ Some medications for anxiety can affect medical conditions, and can interact with other medications, including herbal products and over-the-counter medications. They may also interact with alcohol and other drugs.

+ Some medications for anxiety are difficult to discontinue, and may trigger uncomfortable symptoms when you reduce the dosage too quickly.

Deciding Whether to Take Medications

The decision of whether to take medications should be made in consultation with your doctor. You should take into account the costs and benefits described in this section. Your doctor can help determine to what extent each is relevant to you. Things like side effects or drug interactions will vary widely among different patients.

You need to consider your own preferences too. Your expectations about a particular treatment can have a big impact on whether it helps. So if you're confident that medication will be useful, you'll be more likely to benefit from it than if you believe that medications probably won't help.

Stages of Medication Treatment

There are five main stages in medication treatment: (1) assessment, (2) initiation, (3) acute treatment, (4) maintenance, and (5) discontinuation and dose reduction.

Assessment

During the assessment phase, your doctor will ask questions to determine the nature of your anxiety problem and to identify the best possible treatment options. He or she will ask about your past treatments and about any details that may influence the decision about which medication to choose. The assessment may also include a physical exam, blood work, and other tests to make sure there are no medical conditions that contribute to your anxiety problems or that may interfere with your anxiety treatment.

Initiation

Medication treatments for anxiety are usually started at a low dosage and increased gradually, referred to as *titration*. Depending on the specific medication and the side effects experienced early in treatment, titration may occur slowly or more quickly. During this phase, you need to be in regular contact with your doctor to keep close track of any complications or side effects, which often emerge early in treatment if they're going to be an issue.

Acute Treatment

The acute treatment phase refers to the period when the medication is at the right dosage to reduce the anxiety symptoms. It's during this time that most of the improvement tends to occur. This phase of treatment usually lasts several months. Your doctor will adjust the dosage as needed to keep side effects under control, and switch medications if side effects prove unmanageable or if the treatment isn't working well enough.

Maintenance

Once symptoms improve, patients usually continue to take the medication for a period of time to maintain the gains made during the acute treatment phase. This is the maintenance phase. In the case of antidepressants (the most commonly prescribed medications for anxiety), the maintenance phase usually lasts a year or longer. For some individuals, this phase can last for many years.

Discontinuation and Dose Reduction

Your doctor may have you discontinue a drug that's not working and either try another drug or turn to a completely different approach. Discontinuation may also occur after an effective medication has been used for some time, to see whether improvements can be maintained without it or at a lower dosage (in cases where the dose is reduced but not eliminated). As mentioned earlier, it's important to discontinue medications or reduce dosages under the supervision of your doctor. Several of the medications that are used to treat anxiety can be dangerous when stopped abruptly, leading to panic attacks, insomnia, anxiety, and even seizures.

Strategies for Choosing among Medications

A number of factors go into your doctor's decision, including effectiveness, indications from regulatory agencies, and issues related to safety (such as side effects and interactions with other drugs).

✦ **Research on effectiveness.** Although some medications have been found to work for most anxiety-related problems, others work well only for certain types of anxiety.

Selecting medications should take into account research findings regarding the effectiveness for your particular problem. Also, if you suffer from depression, your doctor would be more likely to select a medication that works for both anxiety and depression rather than one that works for anxiety alone.

✦ **Indications by regulatory bodies.** The marketing and sale of medications are heavily regulated. For example, in the United States, the FDA approves medications for various purposes, or *indications*. In Canada, the agency that approves medications is called the Health Protection Branch (HPB), which is part of Health Canada. To be officially approved by the FDA or the HPB, a medication must be proven safe and effective for the problem it's intended to treat.

Many medications, however, are intended to be used for one problem (such as depression) but also work for anxiety disorders, though they haven't been officially approved for the latter. (This is because it costs many millions of dollars to obtain an FDA indication, and pharmaceutical companies typically don't invest in this process without a high likelihood of making a good return on their investment. Once a medication has been around a while and is available generically, it no longer makes financial sense for a pharmaceutical company to bother seeking new indications.)

✦ **Side effect profile.** Your doctor will aim to recommend a medication with as few side effects as possible, and will pay special attention to side effects that are most likely to be an issue for you. For example, if you already struggle with being overweight, it would be important to select a medication for which weight gain is a less likely side effect. Similarly, if you tend to feel dizzy, your doctor would likely try to find a medication that doesn't list dizziness as a side effect.

✦ **Interactions with other medications.** If you're already taking medications for another condition, your doctor will select an anxiety medication that's unlikely to interact with your other treatments. This includes supplements, over-the-counter medications, and herbal products.

✦ **Interactions with medical conditions.** If you have a medical condition, such as high blood pressure or seizures, your doctor will be sure to bypass the medications for anxiety that could worsen the problem.

✦ **Interactions with recreational drugs.** Medications interact to varying degrees with alcohol and other drugs. You need to let your doctor know about your alcohol or drug use so that the possibility of such interactions can be minimized.

✦ **Pregnancy.** When it comes to treating women who are either pregnant or breastfeeding (or plan to be), some medications are known to be safer than others. Your doctor can take this into account when recommending a medication for your anxiety.

✦ **Previous treatment history.** If you have responded well to a particular medication in the past, your doctor may suggest that medication again. If you responded poorly, your doctor will probably prescribe a different medication.

✦ **Treatment of a family member.** If someone in your family has responded well to a particular drug, your doctor might try the same medication for you. Just as anxiety can run in families, responses to particular medications may also run in families.

✦ **Half-life of the medication.** The half-life of a medication is the length of time it takes for the amount of drug in your bloodstream to decrease to half of its peak level after absorption, as it is broken down by the body. The shorter a drug's half-life, the more frequently you must take the drug to maintain a steady state of medication in your system. Also, a drug with a shorter half-life may be associated with more severe discontinuation symptoms because it's broken down or eliminated more quickly by the body.

Generally, a drug with a longer half-life can be taken less often, poses less of a problem if you forget to take a dose one day, and is easier to discontinue. Drugs with longer half-lives stay in the system longer, however, so it's important not to start a new medication right after stopping an old one. Your doctor will take into account the half-life of a medication before recommending it.

✦ **Cost.** Medications that have been around a while tend to cost less than newer medications because they're more likely to be available in a generic form. If cost is an issue for you, your doctor can take this into account when recommending particular drugs.

As you can see, the process of selecting a medication can be complex—and these are only some of the issues your doctor will consider. Many doctors have their "favorite" medications that they tend to prescribe more frequently because they have more experience with them and are therefore more comfortable recommending them. Doctors are also more likely to prescribe medications that their patients request—all that direct-to-consumer television advertising for medications has had an impact!

Introduction to Effective Medications

As we mentioned, anxiety disorders are treated primarily with antidepressants and anti-anxiety medications, though there are studies supporting a small number of other medications, as well as certain herbal products. In the next few sections, we'll review these treatment options.

Note that an effective medication is not necessarily one that leads to complete elimination of all anxiety symptoms. A small percentage of people will be completely symptom-free by the end of treatment, a small percentage will receive no benefit, and most people will see a significant (but not complete) reduction in symptoms. In other words, it's not unusual to retain some anxiety symptoms after being successfully treated with medication.

There are two main types of studies that are done to evaluate the effectiveness of medications. The first is called an *open trial.* In an open trial, people are given a medication for a period of time, and their symptoms at the end of treatment are compared to their symptoms before treatment began. Both the physician and the patient know what medication is being used and what it's intended to do. Open trials are relatively inexpensive to run (compared to other types of treatment studies), and are often the first step in testing out a medication.

One needs to be very careful when interpreting the findings of an open trial, however. Although positive results may be due to the physical effects of the drug, they may also be due to other factors, including the passage of time (people often start treatment when they are feeling at their worst, and might be expected to improve over time even if they were to receive no treatment at all), a patient's expectations for improving, or the doctor's expectations that the patient will improve (positive expectations by the patient or the doctor can affect the outcome). An open trial tells us whether symptoms have improved by the end of treatment, but it doesn't tell us much about why.

The gold standard for testing the effects of a medication is known as a *randomized controlled trial* (RCT). The term *controlled* means that various other explanations for the results are accounted for, such as the effects of time and the expectations of the patient and prescribing doctor. An example is the placebo-controlled study, in which the drug being studied is compared to a placebo pill that contains no real medication. The term *randomized* means that patients are randomly assigned to receive either medication or placebo. The pills or capsules used for both the real medication and the placebo are identical in appearance, and neither the patient nor the doctor knows which is being taken until the study has ended. (These studies are often referred to as "double-blind" since both patient and doctor are "blind" with respect to which treatment is being received.)

To be considered effective, researchers typically want to see that a drug has been shown in a double-blind RCT to be more effective than placebo. Here's an example of why. A recent study on the use of venlafaxine (an antidepressant) for treating panic disorder found that after 10 weeks on the medication, patients were experiencing an average of about five fewer panic attacks during the last 2 weeks of treatment, compared to the 2 weeks before they started treatment. Sounds pretty impressive ... until you look at the results for placebo. In this study, people taking placebo were experiencing four fewer panic attacks during the last 2 weeks of treatment than during the 2 weeks before the start of treatment. Pretty close! If the placebo condition hadn't been included for the purpose of comparison, the effects of venlafaxine would have seemed more dramatic than they were.

It's not enough to show that people taking a drug improve—they need to have improved more than people taking placebo. Most of the treatments described in this section have been studied in placebo-controlled conditions.

One last thing: information on medications changes quickly. The FDA is continually updating its list of approved medications for various problems. Researchers publish new studies on existing and new medications all the time. So you should supplement the information you learn about particular medications in this chapter with other sources of information, including discussions with your doctor. The Appendix also includes some recommended readings on medication treatments, some of which were our sources for the recommended dosages listed in this chapter.

Antidepressants

The most frequently recommended medications for anxiety disorders are actually officially classified as antidepressants. Don't be misled by the name. In addition to helping people who suffer from depression, these medications also help reduce symptoms of anxiety disorders, and some of them can be used to treat various other problems (such as bulimia, smoking, chronic pain, certain childhood emotional problems, and bed wetting).

Generally, antidepressants take 2–6 weeks to start working once an adequate dose is reached. It's usually recommended that patients continue to take their medications for a year or longer after improving before trying to discontinue them. Relapse rates may be higher if antidepressants are discontinued too early. For most (but not all) of these drugs, discontinuation is fairly easy, and is associated with few uncomfortable symptoms, if any. Again, never discontinue antidepressants without consulting with your prescribing doctor first. In many cases, he or she will recommend that you taper off the medication gradually. In this section, we review the most frequently prescribed antidepressants for anxiety-related problems.

Selective Serotonin Reuptake Inhibitors

For many anxiety disorders, selective serotonin reuptake inhibitors (SSRIs) are the first choice among medications. Table 10.1 includes a list of available SSRIs (both brand names and generic names), as well as the recommended starting and maximum doses for each and the conditions for which the medication has been approved by the FDA. The maximum dosages are recommendations only and are sometimes exceeded.

Note that although different SSRIs have different FDA indications, there is enough evidence to suggest that they're about equally effective in treating most anxiety disorders, including panic disorder, social anxiety disorder, obsessive–compulsive disorder (OCD), posttraumatic stress disorder (PTSD), and generalized anxiety disorder (GAD). The main exception is specific phobias, for which there is little research supporting SSRIs (or any other antidepressants).

SSRIs first appeared in the early 1980s, when fluoxetine (Prozac) was introduced. Escitalopram (Lexapro in the United States, Cipralex in Canada) is the newest SSRI. Although the SSRIs affect our brains in a number of ways, they are believed to make their impact on depression by altering levels of serotonin and by affecting the sensitivity of serotonin receptors in the brain. *Serotonin* is a neurotransmitter that is involved in controlling our emotions as well as other aspects of our psychological functioning (a *neurotransmitter* is a chemical that transmits information from one brain cell to another).

The most common side effects from taking SSRIs include nausea, diarrhea, headache, sweating, anxiety, tremor, sexual dysfunction, weight gain, dry mouth, palpitations, chest pain, dizziness, twitching, constipation, increased appetite, fatigue, thirst, and insomnia. A daunting list! Fortunately, most people experience few (if any) of these symptoms, and they're usually mild in nature. Many of these side effects tend to be worse during the first few weeks of treatment or after a dose increase, so hang in there and the symptoms will probably improve over time. (Some side effects, particularly weight gain and sexual side effects, tend not to improve over time, though, unless the dosage is decreased.) Side effects can be managed by starting SSRIs at a low dosage and

table 10.1. **SSRIs**

Generic name	Brand name (USA/ Canada)	Suggested starting dose	Suggested maximum dose	FDA indications
citalopram	Celexa	20 mg	40–60 mg	Depression
escitalopram	Lexapro/ Cipralex	5–10 mg	20 mg	Depression
				Generalized anxiety disorder
fluoxetine	Prozac	20 mg	80 mg	Depression
				Obsessive–compulsive disorder
				Panic disorder
fluvoxamine	Luvox	50 mg	300 mg	Depression
				Obsessive–compulsive disorder
paroxetine	Paxil	20 mg	60 mg	Depression
				Generalized anxiety disorder
				Obsessive–compulsive disorder
				Panic disorder
				Posttraumatic stress disorder
				Social anxiety disorder
paroxetine CR	Paxil CR	25 mg	62.5 mg	Depression
				Panic disorder
				Premenstrual dysphoric disorder
				Social anxiety disorder
sertraline	Zoloft	50 mg	200 mg	Depression
				Obsessive–compulsive disorder
				Panic disorder
				Posttraumatic stress disorder
				Premenstrual dysphoric disorder
				Social anxiety disorder

increasing them gradually to give your body a chance to get used to the medication. In people with anxiety problems, the starting dose may be even lower than the official recommended starting dose.

Generally, SSRIs are relatively easy to discontinue. An exception is paroxetine (Paxil), which has a very short half life and should be discontinued slowly. If paroxetine is stopped suddenly, or if doses are missed even for a few days, an individual is likely to experience symptoms such as sleep problems, anxiety, nausea, diarrhea, dry mouth, vomiting, sweating, and other uncomfortable feelings.

Selective Serotonin and Norepinephrine Reuptake Inhibitors

Selective serotonin and norepinephrine reuptake inhibitors (SNRIs) act on two different neurotransmitter systems in the brain: serotonin and norepinephrine. There are currently two available SNRIs: venlafaxine and duloxetine. The extended release formula of venlafaxine (Effexor XR) is the best studied SNRI for anxiety. There are double-blind, placebo-controlled studies supporting the use of this medication for treating a number of anxiety disorders, including social anxiety disorder, panic disorder, GAD, and PTSD. Research also shows that venlafaxine XR leads to similar improvements in OCD as paroxetine (an SSRI that is FDA-approved for OCD).

Duloxetine is a more recently introduced SNRI. There is much less research on its use for anxiety. For the time being, there is evidence from well-controlled studies supporting the use of duloxetine for the treatment of GAD, but no research on the use of this medication for other anxiety disorders, except for a few case studies. Duloxetine is available in the United States, where it now has an FDA indication for GAD, and has recently been approved in several other countries, including Canada.

Table 10.2 provides some summary information on the SNRIs, including therapeutic dose ranges and FDA indications. SNRIs typically take 1–4 weeks to kick in once an adequate dose is reached. Common side effects include constipation, loss of appetite, nausea, dry mouth, dizziness, insomnia, nervousness, sexual dysfunction, sleepiness, sweating, and weakness, among others. SNRIs, particularly venlafaxine, should be stopped gradually after prolonged use to avoid uncomfortable discontinuation symptoms.

Noradrenergic/Specific Serotonergic Antidepressant

The only noradrenergic/specific serotonergic antidepressant (NaSSA) available is a medication called mirtazapine (Remeron). Like the SNRIs, mirtazapine affects both norepinephrine and serotonin levels in the brain. Although this drug is approved by the FDA solely for the treatment of depression, preliminary findings (mostly from small uncontrolled studies) suggest that it may be an effective treatment for social anxiety disorder, panic disorder, PTSD, and OCD. There is insufficient research, in the form of large placebo-controlled trials, to firmly establish the effectiveness of mirtazapine for treating anxiety. Table 10.2 shows recommended doses. Some of the more common side effects include weight gain, constipation, dry mouth, sleepiness, and blurred vision.

table 10.2. **SNRIs and NaSSA**

Generic name	Brand name (USA/ Canada)	Suggested starting dose	Suggested maximum dose	FDA indications
SNRIs				
venlafaxine XR	Effexor XR	37.5–75 mg	225 mg	Depression
				Generalized anxiety disorder
				Panic disorder
				Social anxiety disorder
duloxetine	Cymbalta	20 mg	40–60 mg	Depression
				Diabetic peripheral neuropathic pain
				Generalized anxiety disorder
NaSSA				
mirtazapine	Remeron	15–30 mg	60 mg	Depression

Tricyclic Antidepressants

This class of medications first appeared in the 1950s, with the introduction of a drug called imipramine. Although there are more than a dozen tricyclic antidepressants, the two that have been studied most extensively for the treatment of anxiety-related problems are imipramine and clomipramine. Table 10.3 provides a summary of these medications, including dosing recommendations and official FDA indications.

Imipramine has been found to be an effective treatment for panic disorder in numerous studies. There is also evidence supporting imipramine for the treatment of PTSD and GAD. It doesn't seem to provide much help for OCD, social anxiety disorder, or specific phobias, however.

Clomipramine is an effective treatment for OCD and panic disorder, but not for specific phobias. Clomipramine has not been studied as a treatment for social phobia, PTSD, or GAD.

Side effects differ among the various tricyclic antidepressants, but tend to include dry mouth, constipation, blurred vision, sedation, sexual dysfunction, sweating, and dizziness. Side effects and potential health risks tend to be more problematic with tricyclic antidepressants than with the newer classes of antidepressants, so they're prescribed less frequently than they used to be.

table 10.3. **Tricyclic Antidepressants**

Generic name	Brand name (USA/ Canada)	Suggested starting dose	Suggested maximum dose	FDA indications
clomipramine	Anafranil	25 mg	200 mg	Obsessive–compulsive disorder
imipramine	Tofranil	25 mg	150 mg	Depression Childhood enuresis (bed wetting)

Other Antidepressants

Phenelzine

Phenelzine (marketed under the name Nardil) is an example of a class of drugs known as monoamine oxidase inhibitors (MAOIs). It has been studied extensively for the treatment of social anxiety disorder, and also has been shown to be effective for the treatment of PTSD and panic disorder. MAOIs are rarely prescribed anymore for anxiety disorders due to their side effects, potential interactions with other medications and medical conditions, and the various dietary restrictions they require. See Table 10.4 for dosing information.

Moclobemide

Moclobemide (marketed under the names Manerix and Aurorix) is a reversible inhibitor of monoamine oxidase-A and, compared to traditional MAOIs, its side effects and interactions are much milder when prescribed in the recommended dose range. A major advantage over the standard MAOIs is freedom from the requirement to restrict foods containing tyramine, such as certain wines, cheeses, and cured meats. It's not available in the United States, but can be prescribed in many other countries, includ-

table 10.4. **Phenelzine and Moclobemide**

Generic name	Brand name (USA/ Canada)	Suggested starting dose	Suggested maximum dose	FDA indications
phenelzine	Nardil	15 mg	90 mg	Depression
moclobemide	Manerix (Canada)	300 mg	600 mg	Not available in the United States

ing Canada. There have been a number of studies on the use of moclobemide in social anxiety disorder, with some showing it to be effective and others finding no differences between this medication and placebo. A recent uncontrolled study found moclobemide to be as effective as the SSRI fluoxetine for treating PTSD following an earthquake.

Moclobemide has not been studied in other anxiety disorders. In Canada, the recommended starting dose for mocobemide is 300 mg, and the official recommended maximum dose is 600 mg—but this medication is often not effective at dosages this low. Clinical experience puts the effective dosage more in the range of 900 mg to as high as 1,500 mg. The problem is that at these dosages, moclobemide acts more like the traditional MAOIs and is associated with many of their risks and side effects. More research is needed to know for sure whether this medication is useful. See Table 10.4.

Reboxetine

Reboxetine (marketed under the names Edronax, Norebox, and several others) increases levels of the neurotransmitter norepinephrine in the brain. It is available in more than 50 countries around the world, but not in the United States or Canada. One preliminary study suggests that this drug may be useful for treating PTSD related to motor vehicle accidents. Another study found reboxetine to be less effective than the SSRI paroxetine for treating panic disorder. More research is needed on the effectiveness of reboxetine for treating anxiety problems.

Bupropion

Bupropion (marketed under the names Wellbutrin and Zyban) increases the amount of the neurotransmitter dopamine (and, to a lesser extent, norepinephrine) in the brain. An advantage of this medication compared to other antidepressants is that it is rarely associated with weight gain or sexual dysfunction. Although bupropion is an effective treatment for depression and for quitting smoking, it does not appear to be helpful for overcoming most anxiety problems, based on the small number of published studies that have assessed it with this in mind. One recent unpublished study, however, found bupropion to be as effective for treating GAD as the SSRI escitalopram.

Anti-Anxiety Medications

Benzodiazepines

Benzodiazepines are considered minor tranquilizers, and their main effect is to slow down the central nervous system. They are most often prescribed as treatments for anxiety, insomnia, seizures, muscle spasms, tension, or alcohol withdrawal. There are more than 15 benzodiazepines available, though only four have been studied extensively for the treatment of anxiety disorders. These are listed in Table 10.5, along with dosing information and FDA indications.

Unlike antidepressants, benzodiazepines work quickly, often within a half hour.

table 10.5. **Benzodiazepines**

Generic name	Brand name (USA/Canada)	Suggested starting dose	Suggested maximum dose	FDA indications
alprazolam	Xanax/Niravam	0.25 mg	1.5–3 mg	Anxiety disorders Panic disorder
clonazepam	Klonopin/Rivotril	0.25 mg	4 mg	Seizure disorders Panic disorder
diazepam	Valium	2.5 mg	10 mg	Anxiety disorders
lorazepam	Ativan	0.5 mg	3–4 mg	Anxiety disorders

Therefore, they can be taken soon before entering an anxiety-provoking situation. But many anxiety experts recommend taking a regular daily dose. Alprazolam and clonazepam have been studied mostly for the treatment of panic disorder and social anxiety disorder, whereas lorazepam and diazepam have been studied mostly for the treatment of GAD. There is little evidence supporting the use of benzodiazepines for OCD or the core symptoms of PTSD. Although there isn't much research on the use of these drugs for specific phobias, doctors sometimes prescribe them for people with this form of anxiety. For example, some people with flying phobias take a benzodiazepine before a flight.

Common side effects of benzodiazepines include sleepiness, lightheadedness, confusion, dizziness, unsteadiness, depression, headache, insomnia, and nervousness. These drugs may also interfere with your ability to drive safely or to operate machinery. Benzodiazepines interact strongly with alcohol, so you can't drink alcohol when taking these drugs. Older adults should use caution when taking benzodiazepines because higher dosages have been associated with an increased likelihood of falling.

One disadvantage of benzodiazepines is that they can be difficult to discontinue. Stopping these drugs abruptly can trigger intense anxiety, panic attacks, insomnia, and even seizures. Withdrawal symptoms are worse when they've been taken at higher dosages and for longer durations. It's extremely important to discontinue these medications very gradually, under the supervision of your doctor. Because of the difficulty of discontinuing them, these drugs are typically not the first choice for long-term treatment of anxiety-related problems. Nevertheless, they are relatively safe when used properly, and most people who want to come off these drugs are able to do so as long as the dosage is decreased gradually.

There is also preliminary evidence that combining a benzodiazepine with an SSRI antidepressant early in treatment can be a useful strategy for certain anxiety problems.

Because SSRIs and other antidepressants usually take a few weeks to start working, the addition of a benzodiazepine during the first month of treatment may lead to improved outcomes early on. After the first month, there's probably little benefit to continuing both treatments, and the benzodiazepine can be discontinued gradually. The benefits of combining a benzodiazepine with an SSRI during the first month of treatment have been investigated in panic disorder and social anxiety disorder. But the number of studies is small, and more research is needed.

Buspirone

Buspirone (marketed under the name Buspar) is a medication approved by the FDA for reducing anxiety symptoms. It's neither a benzodiazepine nor an antidepressant. Like the antidepressants, buspirone takes a few weeks to start working. Research supports the use of buspirone for treating GAD, but it hasn't been found to be effective for treating other anxiety problems. The recommended starting dosage is 5 mg per day, with a suggested maximum of 30 mg per day. Side effects tend to be mild, and may include dizziness, lightheadedness, headache, nausea, sweating, and nervousness.

Anticonvulsants

Anticonvulsants are used for treating seizure disorders, but there's evidence that certain ones may help with anxiety too. In fact, all the benzodiazepines discussed earlier have anticonvulsant properties. There is preliminary evidence supporting the use of two other anticonvulsants for treating anxiety: gabapentin (Neurontin) and pregabalin (Lyrica). Gabapentin has been found to be more effective than placebo in a study on social anxiety disorder and another on panic disorder. Placebo-controlled trials have shown pregabalin to be an effective treatment for GAD and, to a lesser extent, social anxiety disorder.

More research is needed to determine how effective these medications are compared to more established options. The recommended starting dose for pregabalin is 150 mg, with a maximum daily dose of 600 mg. Gabapentin is often started at 300 mg daily and may be increased up to 1,800 mg daily. Common side effects of these medications include drowsiness, dizziness, and unsteadiness.

Beta-Adrenergic Blockers

Beta-adrenergic blockers (or "beta-blockers") are typically used to treat high blood pressure. They also can reduce some of the physical symptoms associated with anxiety, such as shaky hands and racing heart. A number of studies have found beta-blockers to alleviate anxiety symptoms in performers, and they're sometimes used by actors, musicians, and public speakers to reduce stage fright. These studies were all conducted with people who did not necessarily have a full-blown anxiety disorder, however.

In studies of people with broader, more generalized social fears (such as fears of meeting new people, dating, conversations, being the center of attention), beta-blockers don't seem to be all that helpful. Nor is there evidence supporting these medications for other types of anxiety problems. They may be useful for specific performance fears, though. The most frequently studied beta-blocker for treating performance anxiety is propanolol (Inderal), which is normally taken in a single dose of 5 to 10 mg, about a half hour before a performance.

Antipsychotic Medications

Antipsychotic medications are primarily used to treat severe mental illness such as schizophrenia. Much of the recent research on these drugs has focused on what are known as second-generation antipsychotics, which include drugs such as risperidone (Risperdal), clozapine (Clozaril), quetiapine (Seroquel), olanzapine (Zyprexa), ziprasidone (Geodon), and aripiprazole (Abilify). In addition to treating schizophrenia, there is now evidence that these drugs may also help with severe mood problems such as bipolar disorder (manic-depression) or treatment-resistant depression, and certain symptoms associated with dementia (for example, agitation in patients with Alzheimer's disease). Occasionally, these medications are also prescribed for anxiety disorders.

Note that much of the research on the use of these drugs for anxiety has involved small studies, often with methodological limitations that make it difficult to draw any firm conclusions. Furthermore, only a few studies have investigated whether these drugs are effective for treating anxiety problems on their own; many of them have focused on combining these medications with other drugs (for example, SSRIs) for individuals with severe anxiety who haven't responded to other treatments. A number of studies on treatment-resistant PTSD and OCD have found improved outcomes when combining a second-generation antipsychotic with another medication (such as an antidepressant or anti-anxiety drug). Not all antipsychotics appear to work equally well, however, and findings from studies are sometimes inconsistent.

In summary, antipsychotic medications may be a useful option for some individuals with certain anxiety problems, such as OCD or PTSD. But they should not be considered until several other treatments have been tried first.

Combining Medications with Psychological Approaches

Since CBT and medications are both effective treatments for anxiety, you might think that the combination of these approaches would be even better, right? A number of studies have examined just this question. Surprisingly, combined treatments seem to be no more effective than either approach on its own, especially over the short term. On average, people are equally likely to improve following treating with medication, CBT, or a combination of the two. But there are exceptions, so that doesn't mean that a combined approach won't be best for you.

Little is known about whether medication, CBT, or combined treatments work best in the long term, once all treatments have been stopped. Panic disorder is the only anxiety problem for which this issue has been studied in well-designed, controlled trials, and the results have varied.

Questions and Concerns about Medications

What follows is a list of questions you might have if you're taking medication for your anxiety, or considering it. The answers depend on the specific medication, of course, as well as on each individual. These are just suggestions of things you may want to discuss with your doctor.

Questions to Ask Your Doctor

✦ "How long will it take for my medication to start working?"

✦ "What can I do if my medication isn't working?"

✦ "What if I forget to take a pill? Should I double up next time?"

✦ "What can I do if I'm experiencing uncomfortable side effects?"

✦ "I have gained a lot of weight lately. Could it be because of my medication?"

✦ "Is it okay to start taking an herbal product along with my medication?"

✦ "Does my medication interact with other drugs I'm taking?"

✦ "Will the medication be safe to take if I have a medical issue [for example, high blood pressure]?"

✦ "I'm thinking about becoming pregnant. Can I continue taking my medication?"

✦ "Is it safe to drink alcohol while on my medication? If so, how much?"

✦ "When is the best time to try reducing the dosage of my medication?"

✦ "If I want to stop my medication, how much time will it take to do it?"

✦ "How long after stopping my medication must I wait before starting something new?"

Herbal Remedies and Other Complementary Therapies

Alternative and complementary treatments are becoming increasingly popular in our society. In fact, a 2002 survey found that 62% of adults in the United States had used complementary and alternative therapies in the past year for a health concern. Treatments such as aromatherapy, Bach flower remedies, hypnotherapy, massage, nutrition, reflexology, reiki, and yoga have all been used to treat anxiety and stress. And there are many more. The website *www.holisticonline.com* recommends 24 different herbal medicines for treating anxiety disorders and almost 40 other complementary and alternative treatments, including acupuncture, acupressure, homeopathy, hydrotherapy, meditation, nutrition and diet therapy, prayer and spirituality, vitamins and supplements, therapeutic touch, color therapy, and biofeedback.

What does research tell us about the effectiveness and safety of such treatments? In most cases, there is very little or no research on these approaches for treating anxiety. In other cases, the existing research has numerous methodological flaws (such as inappropriate or invalid measures of anxiety, inadequate numbers of participants, poorly described methods, poor controls for expectations by the participant or the investigator, or lack of placebo comparison). Only in a few cases are there well-conducted studies supporting these treatments.

Herbal Remedies

Herbal remedies have been used for centuries by many different cultures to treat anxiety and other emotional difficulties. As we just mentioned, there are few serious studies of their effectiveness. Consumers should also be aware that quality control for herbal products can be uneven. In North America, these substances are not well regulated, and the amount of actual product in each capsule or pill may vary from what is printed on the bottle and from brand to brand. If these products do work (beyond possible placebo effects), they probably reduce anxiety by altering brain chemistry, which means that they may have associated side effects, interactions, and withdrawal symptoms, just like any other medications. Therefore, they should be used with caution. If you are taking medications, inform your doctor of any supplements or herbal treatments that you are using or considering trying.

In a review of studies on eight different herbal remedies for anxiety—blue skullcap (*Scutellaria lateriflora*), gotu kola (*Centella asiatica*), guarana (*Paullinia cupana*), kava (*Piper methysticum*), keenmind (*Bacopa monniera*), lemon grass (*Cymbopogon citratus*), passion flower (*Passiflora incarnate*), and valerian (*Valeriana officinalis*)—the only product that had enough support to conclude that it is an effective remedy for anxiety was kava.

Kava is a social and ceremonial herb from the South Pacific reported to have sedative, anti-anxiety, antistress, and anticonvulsant effects. Chemically, it is believed to act on the gamma-aminobutyric acid (GABA) system (*GABA* is a neurotransmitter in the brain that is involved in anxiety). This is not surprising—benzodiazepines and alcohol also have their effects on the GABA system. Most studies on kava have been in people from the general population rather than people with a specific anxiety disorder. So, although there is evidence that kava can reduce day-to-day anxiety in nonclinical groups, studies in people with GAD have generally found that kava is no more effective than placebo, and there's very little research on its use in treating other specific anxiety problems.

In light of the lack of evidence, as well as recent concerns about possible liver problems, it's probably advisable to avoid kava as a treatment for anxiety disorders.

Another herb that has been studied for anxiety is St. John's wort (*Hypericum perforatum*). St. John's wort is an herbal medicine for which some studies have found a positive effect in the treatment of depression. In studies of both OCD and social phobia, however, St. John's wort was found to be no more effective than placebo. Controlled studies for other anxiety disorders have not been done.

Galphimia glauca is a plant used in Mexican traditional medicine for "calming nerves." A recent double-blind, controlled study investigated the benefits of an herbal product prepared from the extract of this plant, compared to lorazepam (a benzodiazepine) for the treatment of GAD and found both products to be equally effective and safe—though side effects were less of an issue with the herbal extract. There is also preliminary evidence supporting *Ginkgo biloba* special extract EGb 761 (an herbal product used to treat cognitive function in older adults with dementia) as a treatment of GAD. More research is needed to confirm whether *G. glauca* and EGb 761 are useful treatments for GAD or other anxiety disorders.

Limited research has been conducted on a number of other treatments, including aromatherapy), Bach flower remedies (in particular, Rescue Remedy), and homeopathy, but placebo-controlled studies do not provide support for the use of these remedies.

Other Complementary and Alternative Treatments for Anxiety

✦ **Acupuncture.** There is some evidence supporting the use of acupuncture for treating GAD, but the studies have many methodological problems. More research is needed to reach any firm conclusions.

✦ **Inositol.** Inositol is a variant of glucose (a simple sugar) that occurs naturally in the body and that can also be taken in supplement form. Preliminary data from controlled studies suggest that this product may be helpful for treating panic disorder and OCD, though more research is needed.

✦ **Meditation.** As noted in Chapter 9, mindfulness meditation can be a useful strategy for managing anxiety and stress. Recent evidence supports the use of acceptance- and meditation-based strategies as a treatment for GAD, though once again, more research is needed.

✦ **Omega-3 fatty acids.** Although there are some reports that omega-3 fatty acid supplements can be helpful in depression, a placebo-controlled study in OCD did not find any differences between omega-3 and placebo. This product has not been studied in other anxiety disorders.

✦ **Therapeutic touch.** There are no randomized controlled trials of therapeutic touch for anxiety disorders.

✦ **Yoga.** Although there are some promising results, most studies have a number of methodological limitations, making it difficult to conclude whether yoga is helpful for anxiety.

That concludes the main part of the program to overcome your anxiety issues. Congratulations—you've learned a lot of strategies for dealing with your anxiety. In Part III we move on to a discussion of how you can change any problem habits and surmount obstacles to treatment so that you can gain—and keep—control over your anxiety for life. The last chapter is a guide for you to share with your family and friends as you go through treatment.

PART III

In the Long Run

II

Creating an Anti-Anxiety Lifestyle

If you're still having trouble with anxiety after trying the techniques in previous chapters, then it may be that particular habits or lifestyle issues are getting in the way. This chapter will help you identify and change these problem areas so you can get back on track and help keep your anxiety from returning.

It's all about the brain. Just like the rest of your body, your brain needs your heart to receive blood. It needs blood to receive oxygen from your lungs and nutrients from the food and liquids you eat and drink. In fact, your brain requires more energy than any other part of your body. So if you start doing things that aren't good for your body—eating unhealthy foods; avoiding physical exercise; sleeping poorly; overusing alcohol, nicotine, and other drugs—your brain is likely to suffer. It dislikes your bad habits as much as the rest of your body does.

In this chapter you'll learn about the relationship between anxiety and five main areas concerning healthy living: diet and nutrition; social life; physical exercise; caffeine, nicotine, alcohol, and other drugs; and sleep.

Diet and Nutrition

The human body is, in a sense, a machine—granted an incredibly sophisticated one—but still a machine. And every machine runs on some sort of fuel. The better the fuel, the better the machine will run. The more sophisticated the machine, the higher quality the fuel it requires. That's why the owners of most cars can get away with using regular unleaded gasoline, but the owners of expensive foreign sportscars may need to use ultrapremium unleaded gasoline. Drivers on professional racing teams often use superefficient racing fuels that aren't even available to the general public.

What does this have to do with anxiety? Our body, including the brain, is like an unbelievably advanced race car. If we give it garden-variety fuel, it will cough, sputter, and run poorly. If we give it superior fuel, it will work better. And when our body works well, our mind works well.

Several recent studies have shown the importance of diet in handling anxiety. In one of the largest surveys ever conducted about mental health in the United States, researchers found that people with anxiety disorders had a 25% greater chance of being obese. Another study conducted at Massachusetts General Hospital found a relationship between anxiety disorders and high cholesterol levels. While these studies don't show that obesity and high cholesterol *cause* anxiety, scientists in England have shown that changes in diet and lifestyle can improve your anxiety as much as regular treatment from your physician.

Most countries make free expert guidelines about healthy diets available to the public. In the United States, for example, the Department of Agriculture has the Food Pyramid (*www.mypyramid.gov*). Canada has established the Canada Food Guide (*www.hc-sc. gc.ca/fn-an/food-guide-aliment/index_e.html*). Both give very useful recommendations for healthy eating. And despite what some people assume, these guidelines don't limit our diets to tofu squares and wheatgrass shakes! They suggest balanced diets, which can include meats, fruits and vegetables, grains and cereals, milk and dairy products, and yes, even sweets or desserts in moderation.

Some people feel that eating this kind of balanced meal would be too expensive. Others think they don't have the time to prepare it, or aren't good enough cooks. Still others believe that they need to skip meals or eat only one type of food to lose weight. Are they right?

✦ **"I can't afford those groceries."** This may seem to be the case, but it usually isn't true—especially if you take the time to shop smart. That frozen chicken dinner may seem cheaper to buy than picking up some fresh chicken, vegetables, and potatoes, but more often than not you're paying extra to have the manufacturer prepare it for you.

✦ **"I don't have the time to prepare or cook balanced meals."** Yes, it takes much less effort to pick up some fast food at the drive-through or to put a frozen dinner in the microwave for 3 minutes than it does to prepare a gourmet meal. But you don't need to make a gourmet meal. A burrito from a box may take only 3 minutes to microwave, but peeling a banana or putting some turkey, tomato slices, and lettuce between two slices of bread takes about the same amount of time.

But we can't survive on turkey sandwiches and bananas alone. And even if we could, we'd be incredibly bored with them inside of a couple of days. Fortunately, lots of television shows and cookbooks show you exactly how to make quick easy meals that are healthy and delicious. It may still take a bit longer than packaged foods, but the extra few minutes will make a huge difference in the health of your body and mind.

Lastly, don't forget about leftovers. Eating healthy home-cooked meals doesn't mean you have to cook every single day. Healthy meals are still healthy when they're reheated a couple of days later! Getting back to the issue of cost, it's usually very economical to make a large dish that you can eat two or three times during the week.

✦ **"I'm a terrible cook. I can't make healthy meals."** Who said you had to be a world-class chef? Start with easy dishes and build up your repertoire. Watch a cooking show. Buy a simple cookbook. Or find a family member or friend who is a good cook and make a deal: you'll buy the groceries if he or she will show you how to cook a favorite dish.

✦ **"I shouldn't eat those meals. I need to lose weight."** First, you need to ask yourself if you really need to lose weight. Don't buy into societal pressures to be overly thin. Many people who are at a healthy weight believe that they should be thinner.

If you truly need to drop some weight, most experts agree that simply eating *less* is not as good as eating *better.* Instead of just consuming fewer calories, try eating balanced meals that are lower in calories. Balanced, healthy meals can be low in calories and fat and still provide excellent nutrients, boost your energy, and actually make your body (that machine we were talking about) run more efficiently. In the long run this will be much better in helping you lose weight and will keep your body and mind healthier.

This isn't to say that we can't splurge every now and then. People with the calmest and most anxiety-free minds will sometimes have a slice of chocolate explosion cake with chocolate icing and chocolate sprinkles. Elite athletes have been known to have a bacon double cheeseburger on occasion. Don't feel that you have to give up the foods you love. The goal is to help your body and mind run a little more smoothly by giving them better fuel *most* of the time.

Social Life

Anxiety can be a very isolating condition. You may fear being around others; sometimes it just feels better to stay home, where you feel safest.

This may be the saddest and most ironic thing about having an anxiety disorder because social support is one of the strongest protective barriers against psychological and emotional problems. If anxiety around other people is a problem for you, we strongly encourage you to review Chapters 5 and 6 and to make social activities a priority on your Exposure Plan. The only way to feel more comfortable around people is to practice it.

But what if you don't have many friends or opportunities to socialize? Here are some helpful pointers for developing new social supports and reconnecting with old friends.

Making New Friends and Social Supports

As anybody who has moved to a new city can tell you, it can be hard to make new friends. It's becoming much rarer these days for neighbors to come over with a casserole or to have a complete stranger strike up a conversation with you at the coffee shop. New friends don't just show up when you need them. You have to actively seek them.

Tip 1: Put Yourself in Places Where Potential Friends Might Be.

Strong friendships usually grow out of shared interests. Occasionally you may come across two friends who are very different, but this is rare. We don't know too many animal rights activists who are friends with hunters, do you? It can be very hard to maintain friendships when two people have very different values or interests. Shared interests could be a common love of cooking, playing sports, quilting, gardening, reading crime novels, singing, or anything else that can help forge a bond between two people.

What are some activities or hobbies that you would enjoy doing, even if you weren't doing them with a friend? Fill in the list.

Things I Enjoy Doing

_____

_____

_____

_____

Look over your list. Can you think of places where you could put into practice some of these activities or hobbies? Are these places that might put you amid people who share your interests and hobbies?

Carol's story provides a good example of how this can be done. Carol was a 35-year-old woman who had had panic attacks and agoraphobia for much of her adult life. Because of her anxiety and panic attacks, she had always found it difficult to go out and to be around people. Even in college, she usually stuck to herself and stayed in her dorm room. As a result, she had no close friends and almost never went out on dates. She eventually worked up the courage to overcome her anxiety and began sessions with a cognitive-behavioral therapist. After about 3 months of therapy, she was virtually free from panic attacks and much more able to go out to crowded or busy places.

Next, she wanted to start working on building up friendships, which she had avoided for most of her life. Carol's therapist encouraged her to generate a list of things she would enjoy doing. The first idea that Carol wrote down was "cooking." She enjoyed watching cooking shows on TV, and she often fantasized about how nice it would be to host a big dinner party. Carol was a fairly good cook, even when she was cooking only for herself. She thought it would be fun to have a friend who shared this interest.

So Carol and her therapist started thinking about places she could go that would put her around people who also enjoy cooking. She remembered that several of the grocery stores in her area offered cooking classes. So did two stores where she sometimes shopped for cookware. After a little searching, she also found adult education programs that offered a number of classes for cooking different styles of food. Finally, much to her surprise, she discovered that not far from her own neighborhood was a dinner club: every month a different person would host a dinner party for the other club members.

Carol started by signing up for one of the adult ed cooking classes, where she learned to cook Chinese food. Though she didn't make any friends that time, she did have fun cooking and being around other people. After taking a few more classes, she started to get to know some of the "regulars" who also enrolled in multiple classes. Eventually, they decided to put their new cooking skills to the test, and Carol invited a few of them over for a potluck dinner.

Carol had a very nice time and felt that these people were becoming her good friends. Buoyed by this experience, she went to the community center and signed up for the neighborhood dinner club. She later said that this was one of the best experiences of her life, as she made friends with many of the people and families in her area. Now Carol goes running in the morning with a small group of these neighbors, including an attractive single lawyer who recently moved into a condo down the street.

Tip 2: Allow New Friendships to Grow Naturally.

Like any relationship, friendships take time to develop. Occasionally you may hear of two people who became best friends almost instantly, but that's pretty rare. More commonly, friendships grow over time.

An interesting way to think about friendships is to look at them like a pyramid. Your best or closest friends would be on the top of the pyramid, and casual acquaintances at the bottom.

Notice how much larger the bottom of the pyramid is than the top. It's typical to have a lot of people we consider casual acquaintances, fewer people we consider friends, even fewer who are close friends, and fewer still who are our best friends.

In most cases, friends move up the pyramid one step at a time. Allow people you meet to start as acquaintances. As you get to know some of them better, you might start to consider them friends. Eventually some of them may become good friends. If you and the other person are lucky, that person may become one of your closest friends. This process usually should go one step at a time. Forcing someone up the pyramid too quickly can backfire. That's what happened to Stewart, who enjoyed someone in his new group of card-playing friends so much that he started calling him several times a week. His new friend didn't have enough time to grow into a close friend and felt bombarded by the constant calls. Now they don't see each other much at all.

Reconnecting with Old Friends

Sometimes people say that they used to have many friends but, when their anxiety problems flared up, the friendships started to dwindle away. This isn't uncommon. As anxiety starts to limit what you can do or where you feel safe going, it creates fewer and fewer opportunities to spend time with your friends. Maybe your friends accommodated your anxiety for a while, but eventually they found it hard always to have to plan around your fears. Maybe you felt ashamed about your anxiety and simply stopped calling old friends. Whatever the case, it's not too late to try to rebuild those friendships.

Reconnecting has an advantage over meeting new friends. When trying to make new friends, you might find that you don't have anything in common with them, you don't like them, or your views or beliefs are not well matched. But when rebuilding an old friendship, you already know that the two of you are compatible as friends.

Keep in mind, however, that rebuilding friendships has some similarities to making new friends. You may find that old friends come back lower on your pyramid than they were before. Give the renewed friendship time to grow, just as you would with new friends.

Physical Exercise

Exercise is a powerful tool for reducing anxiety, as well as stress and depression. In fact, regular exercise for as little 30 minutes a day can have as big an impact on your anxiety as medications or therapy! Exercise is seldom prescribed as part of a treatment plan for anxiety, but now you know it would be a good idea to add it yourself.

We don't know *how* exercise manages to reduce anxiety. It might be due to our brains releasing endorphins (the "happy" brain chemicals that our bodies produce naturally when exercising), changes in other brain chemicals, improvements in our self-image, or just a by-product of getting out and doing things instead of hiding indoors all day.

Whatever the reason, exercise is a great way to reduce anxiety and stress.

How Can I Begin?

Only your physician or an experienced personal trainer can help you decide what exercises would be best for you, given your age, weight, and fitness level. But remember that exercise and fitness aren't just about running marathons or lifting weights at the gym. Going for a brisk walk at the park for 30 minutes can be just as helpful. Healthy exercise programs can be designed for everyone, whether you're already fit or you have problems with excess weight or obesity, medical issues, or even a disability or problems with mobility.

And exercise does not need to be boring! Exercising in group activities is one way to make the process more fun, and it combines the benefits of exercise with the benefits of social activity. Sign up for an aerobics class, play on a recreational soccer team, or join a walking or running club. Find activities that you will enjoy. Needless to say, you'll be much more likely to stick with activities that you find fun than activities that bore you. You will be surprised at how beneficial it is for your physical and mental health.

Exercise or Physical Activities I Might Enjoy

_____

_____

_____

_____

Start off with easier activities and then build up to more strenuous ones. One of the main reasons people quit exercise or fitness routines is that they feel overwhelmed with the plan they have set up for themselves. Someone might decide to go to the gym and lift weights every other day, then find that his muscles are too sore after the first day of heavy lifting. Someone else might want to run 3 miles every morning before work, only to get discouraged when she can only go a mile before becoming exhausted. Keep the plan simple at first and then increase the intensity of your physical activity over time. Plan it all out on Form 11.1. (It's followed by Form 11.2, an example of a filled-in form.)

form 11.1	**Steps to Build Up My Physical Activities**
Activity:	
Eventual goal:	
Intermediate steps:	
Realistic starting point:	

form 11.2	**Steps to Build Up My Physical Activities—Completed Example**
Activity:	Jogging/running
Eventual goal:	Run 3-mile track around the park three times each week Run all 3 miles one time, walk the next time, etc.
Intermediate steps:	Run 2 miles, and walk the last mile Run first mile, walk the other two
Realistic starting point:	Walking (quickly) around the 3-mile track every other day

Form 11.2 is the form completed by Diego, who thought that jogging around the park would be a good activity for him. He thought about playing tennis and going to the gym too, but he wisely decided to hold back and not try to do too much at once.

Caffeine, Nicotine, Alcohol, and Other Drugs

Narcotics, alcohol, nicotine, and even caffeine are drugs. You should take a close look at how these drugs might be influencing, or even causing, your anxiety. In some cases, using one of these substances might be *directly* responsible for a large part of your anxiety. Caffeine is a common example, but not the only one. Other times, people use these substances to help cope with their anxiety, believing that it will help them calm down. This approach may work ... in the short term. As you will learn in the next sections, in the long term it can actually maintain (or even strengthen) your anxiety.

Caffeine

Caffeine is the most widely used drug in the world. It is all around us, in coffee, tea, soft drinks, and even chocolate. We sometimes don't think of it as a drug because it is so commonplace—and because we don't see strung-out "coffee junkies" in back alleys or under bridges. But caffeine is a drug—a stimulant, to be precise. It speeds up our minds and bodies for a relatively short period of time.

Most of the time, caffeine has no negative effects on us. In fact, many people can't imagine their day without drinking a cup of coffee first thing in the morning. If you are dealing with anxiety difficulties, however, it might be wise to start thinking about cutting down or eliminating caffeine from your daily life. Why? Because caffeine can exacerbate your anxiety in three ways.

First, it can trigger an episode of anxiety or panic. This is particularly common among people with panic disorder, who are sensitive to unusual sensations in their bodies. For example, someone with panic disorder might be sensitive to how fast her heart is beating because she interprets it as a sign of an impending heart attack. Since caffeine speeds up the body, including the heart, she might mistake her quickening pulse for a heart attack.

Second, caffeine can amplify your anxiety. Remember, when you're anxious, your body is in that fired-up fight-or-flight mode. Adding a stimulant like caffeine will either keep your body in that fired-up state for longer or speed your system up even more.

Finally, in a few unexpected cases, people's anxiety seems almost completely due to drinking too much caffeine. By slowly cutting back on caffeine use, they find that their anxiety and restlessness go away almost completely.

If you choose to reduce your caffeine, keep in mind that caffeine is an addictive drug. Your body gets used to it, and some people will have withdrawal problems (usually headaches) and cravings if they stop suddenly. Reduce your caffeine levels gradually. This may mean cutting back by one cup of coffee or can of cola each day, or replacing some of your coffee or cola with noncaffeinated alternatives. Some people find that drinking "half-caff" coffee (half regular and half decaffeinated coffee) helps them cut back.

Alcohol

Alcohol, a *depressant* drug, can suppress feelings of anxiety in the short term, which is probably why people with anxiety disorders have elevated rates of heavy drinking and alcoholism. In fact, some studies show that about one in five people with an anxiety disorder abuses alcohol, which is more than twice the rate of alcohol use disorders in the general public.

Though alcohol can reduce anxiety in the short term, in the long term it can make anxiety worse, especially for people who have panic attacks. After a person drinks alcohol, his or her body goes through a period of "rebound" during which it recovers from the episode of drinking. This not only brings on the experience of a hangover but it can increase the chance of anxiety and panic attacks. Second, and more important, using alcohol to drown out anxiety can prevent you from overcoming your anxiety. It can also increase the anxious feelings.

This is what happened to Eric, who suffered from social anxiety. He was always anxious that other people were thinking negatively about him. He feared that he would do or say things that would embarrass or humiliate himself. He eventually found that a little "liquid courage," as he called it, helped him feel more at ease when he was around people. After a while, however, Eric started to believe that he *needed* a drink to be able to be around others. So when he did have an enjoyable social encounter, he came to believe that it was *because* he had been drinking. Eric believed that the alcohol protected him from other people laughing at him and thinking he was stupid. By drinking whenever he socialized, Eric never had the opportunity to learn that this wasn't true.

If this sounds familiar, it may be because there was a similar discussion in Chapter

5 in the section on false-safety behaviors. These are the things we sometimes do, such as washing hands, checking locks, or keeping a cell phone handy, to ward off anxieties. Alcohol is one of the most common false-safety behaviors. Like any false-safety behavior, it prevents you from learning that the situations and objects that trigger your anxiety aren't as dangerous as you think. Instead, the anxious mind mistakenly learns that the bad consequences you expected were prevented because of the alcohol.

Finally, alcohol can make anxiety worse, especially if a person drinks to the point of becoming drunk. Eric would start slurring his words and acting silly when he had too much to drink. Occasionally, he would be unable to recall parts of his evening. This would make him very anxious because he was sure that people had seen how drunk he was and thought he had been acting like an idiot. Sometimes this was indeed what had happened. Once during a business dinner with a client, he made a few inappropriate comments because of his drinking and almost lost an important contract.

If you feel you use alcohol as a way to manage your anxiety, you really should talk to a professional who can help you either get your drinking under control or stop it altogether. You might just need to make a conscious effort to stop using alcohol when you feel anxious. Or you might require some form of treatment for excessive alcohol use. If you need it, please have a qualified professional such as a physician or psychologist help you assess your drinking honestly. A professional can also recommend appropriate treatment options.

Nicotine

Nicotine is one of the main drugs found in cigarettes, cigars, pipe tobacco, and chewing tobacco. Many people don't know that nicotine is actually a *stimulant* drug, like caffeine. People may say that they smoke a cigarette to relax, but in their bodies quite the opposite is happening. Smoking, in fact, keeps the body fired up, and there is strong evidence of a relationship between smoking and anxiety problems.

If you smoke, you should also think about how the health risks of smoking might be affecting your fears. If your anxiety revolves around fears of health problems, is your use of tobacco contributing to those fears? If shortness of breath is a trigger for your anxiety, is your smoking making this condition worse? All smokers know that smoking is an unhealthy habit and that they should try to quit. But smokers with an anxiety disorder also need to consider how the nicotine may be affecting their anxiety.

Drugs, Narcotics, and Abused Medications

Some people with anxiety disorders use drugs, much like alcohol, as a way of trying to cope with the anxiety. But, like alcohol, drugs can ultimately contribute to the anxiety problem. Some drugs do this directly. Cocaine, for example, can cause people to have particularly severe panic attacks. Hallucinogenic drugs like LSD can create terrifying experiences that feed your fears. Even prescription or over-the-counter medications can have bad anxiety side effects when used excessively or improperly.

If you are using any illicit drugs, or if you feel you are using prescription or nonprescription medications in a way that is excessive, you really need to discuss this issue with a professional. This might be your physician, a psychologist or other mental health professional, a member of the clergy, or anyone else with professional training who can help you. Drug use is a serious problem for anyone in the general population; for someone with an anxiety disorder, it could be especially disastrous.

Sleep and Anxiety

Finally, we turn our attention to sleep. Does your anxiety interfere with the amount of sleep you're getting? Does it affect the quality of your sleep? If so, you are not alone. Up to two thirds of people who seek treatment for an anxiety disorder also complain about insomnia. Worrying at night, panic attacks that wake you from your sleep, and even nightmares about traumatic events can all get in the way of getting a good night's sleep.

Fortunately, as you begin to overcome your anxiety problems, your sleep will begin to improve. But there are some strategies you can use to help get your sleep back on track right now. This is important because emerging research indicates that poor sleep quality can make you even more vulnerable to experiencing anxiety and the negative effects of stress. Health professionals and sleep specialists refer to these techniques as "sleep hygiene."

The strategies that make up sleep hygiene are simply a set of good sleeping habits that we sometimes forget. If you're having problems sleeping, see if anything in the following list helps you get to sleep and stay asleep:

1. Get on a regular bedtime schedule. Although sleep is partly controlled by a biological cycle, it's also partly habit. Your body can become "trained" to start the sleep cycle at a certain time and to wake at a certain time. This is why experts in child development and parenting stress the importance of setting (and sticking to) strict bedtime routines for children. It may take some time to get used to it, but setting yourself a firm time to go to sleep and making yourself get up 8 hours later can be one of the most important factors in reestablishing your sleep patterns.

2. Wake up at a set time each day. If you have trouble falling asleep, it may be tempting to sleep in the next morning. But that will just perpetuate the cycle by making it harder for you to fall asleep that night. If you tend to have insomnia, it's best to force yourself to wake up at a set time (about 8 hours after your scheduled bedtime). You'll be much more likely to fall asleep at night.

3. Avoid sleeping at other times. If developing good sleep habits at night is your goal, then it's essential not to sleep or nap at other times. This often runs against people's intuition: "If I'm not sleeping well at night, why shouldn't I get a nap in when I can?" You shouldn't because it can affect how long you sleep at night. And consecutive hours of sleep are better for you than the same amount of sleep in shorter increments.

4. Stay away from alcohol or caffeine near bedtime. It's surprising how many people with sleep problems forget that caffeine is a stimulant, which will interfere with your sleep. And few people know that alcohol, a depressant, is equally bad for your sleep. Alcohol may make you feel sleepier, but it interferes with rapid eye movement (REM) sleep—the period of sleep during which we dream. REM sleep is an essential phase during which we obtain good restorative sleep.

5. Arrange your sleeping space. Sometimes sleep problems are related to *where* you try to sleep. First, sleep is best on a comfortable bed with good bedding. Avoid sleeping on the sofa or anywhere else that isn't comfortable. Second, minimize light and noises that can keep you awake. This may be difficult if you work nights or live near a train station, but there are still things you can try. Blackout curtains can eliminate almost all light from entering your room, and small foam earplugs are an excellent and comfortable way to minimize noise. Finally, keep the temperature of your bedroom comfortable at night. Rooms that are too hot or too cold can interfere with your sleep.

6. Reserve your bed for sleep only. Okay—sex too! But otherwise, train your body to associate going to bed with sleeping. Remember, sleep is part habit. You want your body to get into the habit of sleeping while in bed. Avoid reading or watching TV in bed, or any other activity that might teach your body that bedtime isn't sleep time. In fact, if you can't fall asleep after about a half hour of trying, it's a good idea to leave your bedroom for a short while rather than lying awake in bed.

7. Practice relaxation. The relaxation skills in Chapter 9 can be used to help you sleep. Practicing relaxation shortly before bed is an excellent way to calm down the mind and body and prepare you to fall asleep.

If you are having sleep problems, give these techniques a try for 2 weeks. The changes may not happen overnight (pun intended), but they will happen with time. Most people find that changing their sleep habits will have a powerful effect on improving their sleep. If your sleep does not improve, speak with your physician or a sleep medicine specialist about other options. He or she can help diagnose whether your sleep problems have a medical cause (such as sleep apnea) and can prescribe medications or other treatments to help you sleep properly again.

Conclusion

This chapter provided you with a host of ideas about how your lifestyle can have a negative impact on your anxiety and how making lifestyle changes can help you in your recovery from anxiety. Some of these lifestyle changes are fairly easy to put into action, while others may be difficult and require assistance from loved ones or professionals.

If you're serious about making some or all of these lifestyle changes, don't try to make them all at once! Breaking habits and changing your lifestyle are tough propositions. Select one area on which to work first and start making those changes. Once you have been able to replace problem lifestyle habits with healthy habits in that area, take a look at another area you want to change. Making changes in a sequential, step-by-step manner is always more effective than trying to change everything about yourself at the same time.

And please, if you're having trouble with alcohol or drugs, talk to a professional. These problems are unlikely to fix themselves, and can lead to serious psychological, medical, and legal issues.

12

Overcoming Treatment Obstacles

This workbook has given you lots of ways to decrease your anxiety. But going from reading a book to making important changes in your life isn't easy. A number of obstacles can get in the way of your anxiety treatment, interfering with your success as you work through the strategies. In this chapter we'll talk about a number of these obstacles and offer solutions for getting around them. As you read through the chapter, you will no doubt find that some sections apply to you more than others. It covers:

+ Difficulty finding the time for treatment
+ Coping with other psychological problems, such as depression or substance abuse
+ Difficulty getting motivated
+ Life stress
+ Medical complications
+ A lack of relevant skills (for example, communication skills, driving skills)

Finding Time

Many of us lead very busy lives and find it hard to squeeze in everything we need to get done. The activities of everyday life—meals, exercising, working, studying, answering e-mails, shopping for groceries, sleeping, taking care of children, socializing, cleaning, paying bills—leave little time for much else. Now we're asking you to find the time to complete diaries, practice exposure, and start implementing other strategies from this book. How can you fit in these new requirements? Here are some suggestions:

+ Remember that the time commitment required for most of the exercises will be temporary. Although treatment is time-consuming, the process of becoming less anxious will not go on forever. The most intensive period of your anxiety treatment will probably last only a few months. Those few months of hard work can translate into a lifetime of keeping your anxiety under control.

✦ **Schedule your homework practices.** We recommend that you schedule your homework practices on a calendar, just as you would any other appointments. If you're planning exposures to overcome a fear of heights, you might block off a period of time from 6:00 P.M. until 7:30 P.M., 5 days per week, to practice being in high places. We have found that people who write their scheduled practices into a calendar are more likely to complete them.

✦ **Make your practices as convenient as possible.** You have to eat each day anyway, so why not make a point of eating with other people if you're afraid of socializing? Similarly, if you fear crowded supermarkets, make sure you do your shopping during peak times instead of when the supermarket is empty. Chances are that many of your exposure practices can occur during activities that you have to do anyway. Can you think of how you might complete some of your homework during the course of your everyday activities so they don't take up much additional time?

You can also take steps to make completing your treatment diaries more convenient. Carry them with you or leave them someplace you can't overlook (on the kitchen table, on your pillow, or the like).

✦ **You don't have to use every single strategy in this book.** If you did, you wouldn't have time for anything else! Changing your anxious thoughts (Chapter 4); exposure to feared situations, thoughts, and feelings (Chapters 5 through 8); practicing relaxation (Chapter 9); and making important lifestyle changes (Chapter 11) all take time. Select the strategies that are most relevant to you and focus on those. Chapter 3 includes information on how to choose the most important strategies for your particular pattern of anxiety.

✦ **Carve out the time you need to practice.** For the first few weeks of your treatment, it may be necessary to reduce some of your other activities to make time to focus on your anxiety. Be realistic, but work your practice into your schedule in the best way for you. If you fear driving, for example, you can either practice an hour every day for an extended period or take a week or two off work and practice driving for several hours each day. Similarly, if you're too busy to practice exposure to heights because you have three young children at home, you might hire a babysitter a couple of times per week (for a few weeks) to free up time for your exposure practices.

✦ **Some practice is better than no practice.** The strategies as described in this book are meant to maximize your chances of success. But if you can't practice as much as we recommend, some is better than none. If practicing exposure five times per week is impossible, try practicing two or three times per week. Your progress may be a bit slower, but chances are that you'll still benefit from the practices.

Coping with Other Psychological Problems

People with an anxiety problem often also suffer from depression, substance use issues, an eating disorder, or problems in their relationships. Depending on their severity, these additional problems may get in the way of overcoming your anxiety. If you suffer from emotional difficulties other than your anxiety, here are some important questions to consider:

✦ **Which problem is causing you the most distress and interfering with your life the most at this time?** If the other difficulty is more severe than your anxiety at the present time, you'll probably need to deal with the other problem first. For example, if your depression is so severe that you can't get out of bed, or if you're thinking about suicide a lot, you need to get treatment for depression first.

✦ **Is the other problem a consequence of your anxiety?** If so, it may make sense to work on your anxiety first. If you feel depressed only from the ways in which your anxiety affects your life, for example, chances are that your depression will improve when your anxiety improves. Work on your anxiety first, especially if the severity of your depression (or other problem) is manageable.

✦ **Is your other problem likely to interfere with your anxiety treatment?** If so, then you should work on the other problem first, or work on it at the same time as your anxiety problem. For example, if you're so depressed that you have no energy to complete your exposure practices, getting treatment for your depression may be necessary before you can fully benefit from them.

✦ **Are you able to put aside your other problems in order to focus on your anxiety?** If not, it may be best to get treatment for your other problems first.

Note that many of the strategies that are useful for overcoming problems with anxiety are also useful for treating other emotional difficulties. People who are depressed often find that their depression improves as they learn to change depressive thoughts, force themselves to do things despite their lack of energy and motivation, and change some of their lifestyle habits (for example, by beginning to exercise regularly).

Also, as you learned in Chapter 10, many of the medication treatments for anxiety also help with depression, as well as other problems. Of course, the focus of this book is your anxiety, but take a look at the Appendix, which includes resources and recommended readings that may be helpful for problems other than anxiety. Seeking professional help for these other issues may also be warranted.

Boosting Your Motivation

We recently asked 35 people who were being assessed in our clinic for possible treatment of obsessive–compulsive disorder (OCD) whether they had any second thoughts about starting treatment for their problem. Almost everyone (33 out of 35 patients, to be exact) reported having some concerns, which fell into four main categories. These are examples of the types of concerns people reported, organized according to these categories. In parentheses, we provide the percentage of people who listed an issue as their top concern.

✦ **Treatment will increase my symptoms (34.3%):**
   —"My obsessions will increase in frequency."
   —"I will develop a new irrational fear."
   —"If I let my guard down, my obsession might come true."
   —"What will I do instead of my rituals?"

✦ **Treatment will fail (28.6%):**
   —"I will be a hopeless case."
   —"I am too severe to change."
   —"I might not be motivated enough."
   —"I might not be strong enough."
✦ **Treatment will succeed (14.3%):**
   —"My personality will change (I will become lazy, careless, and so on)."
   —"Others will be more demanding of me."
   —"People will be mad that I didn't overcome the problem sooner."
   —"I will relapse after treatment ends."
✦ **General treatment concerns (14.3%):**
   —"I fear disclosing myself to strangers."
   —"Treatment is inconvenient—I will have to miss work."
   —"The doctor will think poorly of me."
   —"I have to drive to treatment and I might hit someone on the way."

As you can see, our patients reported all sorts of concerns about seeking treatment, the most common of which were related to fears of their symptoms worsening or of treatment not working. Of course, ambivalence or uncertainty about treatment is not unique to OCD. Do you see yourself in any of these statements? People often feel ambivalent about overcoming their anxiety and other emotional problems they may have. Surely, people who feel anxious want to feel better. Yet there may be a part of them that is afraid to begin treatment.

Experts on motivation believe that three things must be present in order for someone to be motivated to overcome a problem: he or she must be willing, able, and ready. The term *willing* refers to whether change is important to the person. The term *able* refers to whether the person is confident in his or her ability to change. And the term *ready* refers to whether change is a high priority for the person at this time.

So, are you willing, able, and ready for treatment? If you aren't sure, here are some suggestions for improving your motivation:

✦ **Consider the costs and benefits of change.** In Chapter 3, we provided you with examples of possible costs and benefits of changing, and you listed your own examples. If you are ambivalent about changing, this is a good time to review the list you made on page 62.

✦ **Focus on *intrinsic* reasons for change.** Intrinsic reasons for change are those that represent your own personal reasons for wanting to change. Intrinsic reasons for changing have to do with your own values. For example, if you value the ability to do things despite feeling anxiety and fear, that would be an intrinsic reason to change. Similarly, if you believe it's important to overcome your anxiety so you can be a better parent (assuming that good parenting is something you value), that would be an intrinsic reason to change. On the other hand, getting over your anxiety so your partner will stop nagging you is an *extrinsic* (or external) reason for changing.

Not surprisingly, intrinsic reasons are more likely than extrinsic reasons to motivate people to change. As you consider the costs and benefits of changing, pay extra attention to the benefits that are consistent with your own intrinsic reasons for changing.

✦ **Focus on problems that you can change.** If you doubt whether the treatments described in this book will actually help, we recommend that you start by working on some of your more straightforward anxiety issues rather than the challenging ones. Once you have made some small gains, your confidence will likely improve, and you'll feel more ready to tackle some of the bigger issues with the help of this book and perhaps a therapist.

✦ **Involve others in your treatment.** Making a public commitment to change is often more motivating than making a private commitment. In other words, if you let several friends know that you will be practicing exposure to enclosed places on a particular day (or even better, *promise* them that you will do so), you may be more likely to practice than if you keep your plans to yourself. The embarrassment of not following through after making a promise to others may be enough to motivate you to complete the practice.

Another way to involve others is to have one or two close friends or family members provide reassurance or encouragement before you complete your practice. A pep talk before your practice may help you to follow through.

Finally, you can directly involve people in your practices. For example, if you fear being in dark theaters, you can make plans to see a movie with a friend. You may be less likely to cancel if someone else is involved.

✦ **Use basic learning principles to reinforce small steps.** Rewards can be a very powerful method of changing behavior. Just as the promise of a regular paycheck helps motivate people to go to work each day, you can include rewards in your own treatment plan to motivate you to complete your practices. For example, if you enjoy going to movies on the weekends, you can make a commitment to see a movie only after you have completed a certain amount of practice during the week. Here's an example of how Rob used rewards to motivate himself to complete his exposure practices:

> Rob suffered from OCD. He washed his hands more than 50 times per day, and he avoided actions that could contaminate him, including shaking hands, touching money, using public bathrooms, and hugging other people (even his own family). His treatment plan involved spending 1 hour per day over 5 days per week touching various things that he perceived to be contaminated. To motivate himself to complete his homework, he gave $1,000 to his best friend. Each Sunday, his friend returned $100 to him if he completed his homework for the week. If not, the friend was free to spend $100 on whatever he wanted or to donate it to charity. Of course, this technique required Rob to be honest about his progress. By adding the weekly rewards to his treatment plan, Rob found it easier to force himself to do his practices.

Note that these sorts of rewards provide extrinsic reasons for change. While they may be useful, you should also identify intrinsic reasons for changing, as described earlier. Ultimately, you're changing to help you be the type of person you want to be.

Managing Stress

As discussed in Chapter 3, significant life stress can interfere with the outcome of treatment. Such stresses include health problems, relationship conflict, divorce, work stress, unemployment, financial strain, living in a dangerous neighborhood, and experiencing legal problems. Over time, many minor stresses, such as car problems and lost luggage during a vacation, can also take their toll. Even positive life events like getting married, starting an exciting new job, or having a baby can be stressful.

There are a number of reasons why increased stress can have a negative impact on treatment. First, when we are under stress we tend to feel more emotional and vulnerable, and we experience more physical symptoms such as a racing heart, muscle tension, dizziness, and breathlessness. As a result, we're more likely to experience higher levels of fear and anxiety in situations that normally would seem manageable. For example, if you experience mild levels of fear while riding elevators, you may find that your fear of elevators is higher when you have a lot of stress at work. In addition to increasing levels of arousal, stress can also affect anxiety treatment by distracting people's attention from their treatment. If you're consumed by the demands of a new baby or the threat of being laid off at work, it will much more difficult for you to work on your OCD or your anxiety in social situations.

High levels of stress can lead to a worsening of other problems as well. For example, people who get headaches tend to experience more of them when they're under stress. People who are prone to depression, anger problems, eating disorders, or alcohol abuse are at risk for having these problems worsen during or following times of stress.

As discussed in Chapter 3, if the stress you are under is temporary (for example, planning a wedding), it may be best to wait until after it has passed before beginning to work on your anxiety problem. But if your stress is ongoing (for example, raising three children and regularly lacking enough money to cover your rent and other expenses), waiting until the stress has passed may not be a realistic option. Rather, it may be best to try to deal with the stress directly.

There are two main ways of dealing with stress. The first involves trying to reduce or eliminate it, and the second involves changing the way you respond to stress.

Reducing Stress Levels

There are direct steps you can take to reduce or eliminate stress. Examples include:

+ Leaving a stressful job
+ Asking the boss for more flexible hours
+ Reducing your college course load from five courses to four courses per term
+ Leaving an abusive relationship
+ Going for marital therapy to reduce conflict in your relationship
+ Getting treatment for your chronic back pain

People often respond to problems in ways that increase the stress in their lives rather than decrease it. When faced with the stress of a challenging assignment, for example, students will often put off working on it until the night before it's due, thereby compounding their stress. Postponing dealing with stress is an ineffective method of coping, particularly if the stress is unlikely to go away on its own.

An alternative method of solving stressful situations is a structured method of problem solving that is most likely to lead to a solution that works. Essentially, problem solving involves five steps:

1. Identify the problem (or problems). In this first step, the goal is to describe exactly what problem is creating stress for you. Be as specific as possible. If there is more than one problem, treat each one as a separate issue rather than lumping all of your problems together into one big problem.

2. Generate possible solutions. In this step, you should generate as many possible solutions as you can—even bad solutions. This process is called "brainstorming." At this point, don't filter your solutions or judge them (evaluating your solutions should be saved for Step 3). If you were to filter your solutions at this stage, you might miss out on a good idea.

3. Evaluate the solutions you have generated. Now you can examine each solution to decide how practical it is and how likely it is to solve your problem.

4. Select the best solution (or solutions). Select the solution that is most practical, most easy to carry out, and most likely to solve the problem.

5. Implement the selected solution. The last step is to carry out the solution you have decided upon. You may discover that carrying out your plan is associated with additional problems that need to be solved. For example, if your solution to a marital problem is to seek marital counseling that raises two new problems: convincing your partner to go with you and finding a qualified marital therapist. You can use these same problem-solving steps to deal with any new challenges that arise during the process of implementing your solutions.

Form 12.1 can be used to help you practice problem solving. We have included a blank copy as well as a completed example (Form 12.2). Notice in Form 12.2 how an acceptable solution to the problem was generated, thereby leading to a significant reduction in the stress level associated with the situation.

Changing Your Response to Stress

A second way of dealing with stress is to change how you respond to the stress. This is particularly useful when you can't reduce or eliminate a stress. There are a number of approaches you can take to deal more effectively with life stresses so they won't be so upsetting:

Cognitive Strategies

The cognitive strategies discussed in Chapter 4 (in particular, *decatastrophizing*) can be used to deal with stress in your life. Rather than focusing on how terrible a situation is,

Problem-Solving Form

1. Identify the problem (or problems).

2. Generate possible solutions.

3. Evaluate the solutions generated.

4. Select the best solution (or solutions).

5. Implement the selected solution.

Problem-Solving Form—Completed Example

1. Identify the problem (or problems).

I have an important meeting at work in a half hour, and my car won't start. It takes me a half hour to get to work, so I can't possibly be on time for the meeting.

2. Generate possible solutions.

1. Try to start my car again.
2. Call the American Automobile Association (AAA) to see if they can start my car.
3. Call a coworker to see if I can get a ride to work.
4. Call a taxi.
5. Call work to reschedule the meeting.
6. Just stay home and enjoy the day off.
7. Quit my job.

3. Evaluate the solutions generated.

—I can try Option 1, but I need to be prepared with another solution in case my car doesn't start.
—Option 2 won't get me there in time because it will take AAA a while to get to my house.
—My coworker who drives this way would have already left for work, and I don't have his cell phone number, so Option 3 won't work.
—Option 4 would probably get me to the meeting on time (cabs usually arrive within a few minutes), but it would cost me about $30.
—Option 5 would not be a good idea—it took 2 months to come up with a meeting time that worked for everyone.
—Options 6 and 7 are silly—I don't think those would go over well with my boss!

4. Select the best solution (or solutions).

I will try to start the car again, and then call a taxi if it doesn't start. It's not an ideal solution, but it's better than the others. $30 for a taxi is worth not missing the meeting.

5. Implement the selected solution.

I tried to start the car again, but it still didn't work. I called the taxi, and it arrived within 5 minutes. I was about 10 minutes late for the meeting, but everyone was very understanding.

try to shift your focus to how you can cope with the situation. Some questions to ask yourself include:

+ "Would this really be as terrible as it seems?"
+ "How can I get past this stress?"
+ "How can I cope with this?"
+ "Will this situation still matter next week or next month?"
+ "How might someone else think differently about this stressful situation?"

Relaxation- and Meditation-Based Strategies

Relaxation exercises, meditation, and acceptance-based approaches (see Chapter 9) are potentially helpful ways to deal with stress. The recommended readings at the back of this book contain additional resources for those who wish to learn more about these strategies.

Increasing Pleasurable Activities

Everyone needs a break from stress. If you are under a lot of stress, taking the time to do things you enjoy (for example, seeing a movie, going out with friends) is an important strategy for managing stress and reducing its impact on your health.

Healthy Lifestyle Habits

As discussed in Chapter 11, healthy lifestyle habits are also important when dealing with stress. More than ever, it is important when under stress to eat well, seek social support, exercise, get a good night's sleep, and reduce use of caffeine, nicotine, alcohol, and other substances.

Medical Issues and Complications

On occasion, people have medical issues that complicate their treatment. Here are some case examples, with suggestions for how they might be dealt with:

Example 1

Frank is a 70-year-old man who recently had a heart attack. He is significantly overweight, though he has recently started to eat more healthy foods. He constantly worries about having another heart attack and is having panic attacks several times per week. He often mistakes these panic attacks for possible heart attacks. Frank avoids arousing activities like sex and exercise because he fears that getting his heart racing might trigger a heart attack. He also avoids driving and crowds for fear of having a panic attack that might then trigger a heart attack.

Suggestions

The first step is for Frank to figure out if the standard treatment strategies might be appropriate. Cognitive strategies are useful for dealing with unrealistic fears, but less so for dealing with realistic fears. Clearly, some aspects of Frank's fear are realistic. Compared to a younger person of normal weight and with no history of heart disease, Frank's risk of a heart attack is higher. But Frank may be exaggerating the risks in his mind. He needs to ask his cardiologist whether he indeed faces an elevated risk of heart attack with sex and exercise. In most cases, people who have had heart attacks are encouraged to exercise. If Frank discovers that aspects of his anxiety are exaggerated or based on misinformation, then he may find cognitive strategies to be useful. Similarly, as long as his cardiologist confirms that it is perfectly fine for him to become aroused, then gradual exposure to the situations he fears would be fine. Other options to consider include a program for weight loss (to reduce his chances of further heart problems), relaxation- or meditation-based strategies, and medications for anxiety.

Example 2

Beth is a 52-year-old woman whose husband, Mike, was recently diagnosed with untreatable cancer. His doctors estimate that Mike will not survive beyond the next month or two. Beth and her husband have been married for more than 25 years. She is devastated by the news, and fears that neither she nor her children (ages 20 and 24) will be able to cope when Mike dies. She also worries about how she will make ends meet without his salary. She is completely consumed by her anxiety, and feels very guilty about being so focused on herself during a time when her husband needs her support.

Suggestions

Clearly Beth is dealing with a situation that anyone would find anxiety-provoking. When someone is experiencing anxiety that is mostly realistic, the focus should be on identifying strategies for coping. These might include seeking social support to deal with the stress (from friends, family, a support group, or a therapist), using problem-solving strategies to come up with solutions to some of the practical challenges that Beth faces (no longer having her husband's salary, for example), and strategies for managing her arousal levels (relaxation, meditation, exercise, medication, or other methods).

Example 3

David is a 34-year-old man who fears fainting while driving. He had fainted a couple of times in his life (about 10 years earlier), though never while driving. He never did figure out why he fainted. David feels lightheaded when he drives, and prefers to avoid driving whenever possible.

Suggestions

The first step would be for David to have a thorough physical exam to confirm that his actual risk of fainting while driving is low. If it is low, it would make sense for David to practice driving, starting in easier exposure practices (when there is little traffic, with someone else he trusts in the car, and so on), and working his way up to more challenging situations once he has begun to recognize that his chances of fainting are low.

Example 4

Lorraine avoids crowded places because she fears that she might have diarrhea in public. Furthermore, unlike many people who have this fear, she actually does experience diarrhea and she doesn't always make it to a bathroom in time. This happens to her without warning every couple of months.

Suggestions

For many people who fear having diarrhea in public, the chances of this actually happening are very low. Those who do experience diarrhea when anxious almost always make it to a bathroom. When there is no bathroom around, the feeling eventually subsides (suggesting they have control over their diarrhea). In these more typical cases, it is important to challenge the predictions that a diarrhea attack will occur and will be unmanageable. Exposure to public places (especially far away from bathrooms) can also be very helpful.

Lorraine's fear seems much more realistic than the typical case. She does have attacks of diarrhea on a regular basis, they occur without warning, and she often doesn't make it to a bathroom in time. In her case, using safety behaviors to protect her from this threat actually makes sense. For example, she might consider wearing adult diapers, carrying a change of clothing with her, and making sure she knows where the bathrooms are in public places. It would also be important for her to see her doctor to learn why she is having these bouts of diarrhea and to receive medical treatment if necessary. If her diarrhea improves, but her anxiety persists, then it might be time to consider strategies for reducing unrealistic anxiety, including cognitive strategies and exposure.

Example 5

Tara has a fear of blood tests. Like many people with blood and needle phobias, she has a history of fainting when having her blood drawn. She also has very small veins, so it's difficult for the doctor, nurse, or technician to find a vein that is large enough for drawing blood. Tara often ends up with painful bruises on her arm and has to have the blood taken from somewhere else, like her hand or leg.

Suggestions

Tara's fear of blood tests seems realistic. Because of her small veins and the pain she endures during the tests, her fear is different than the more exaggerated fears seen in most people with blood phobia. In Tara's case, it makes sense to try to minimize the pain and bruising by making sure that the person taking her blood is very experienced. It would also be helpful for her to request to have the blood drawn from an area that has worked in the past rather than from her arm. To deal with Tara's fainting, a strategy called "applied muscle tension" can be used. This involves tensing all the muscles of the body during exposure to blood, which temporarily raises the blood pressure and prevents fainting. This procedure is discussed in more detail elsewhere, particularly in *Overcoming Medical Phobias* (Antony and Watling), listed in the Appendix.

Improving Relevant Skills

Sometimes a person's fear makes sense because he or she lacks certain basic skills that are required to be safe in the situation. For example, some people who fear skiing may lack the experience and training to be able to ski safely. They may benefit from some skiing lessons in addition to standard exposure practices.

Two commonly feared situations in which it is helpful to have strong skills include driving and social situations.

Driving Skills

Most people who fear driving actually drive very well. Unlike confident drivers, they rarely speed and they hold the steering wheel with both hands. They don't cut off other drivers, they don't tailgate, and they don't allow themselves to be distracted by eating, putting on makeup, talking on the phone, or reading while driving. They actually drive much more safely than they think they do. Nevertheless, there are some fearful drivers who *should* be afraid because they drive unsafely. Often, these fearful drivers have very little driving experience. An example might be someone who obtained his or her license as a teenager and then spent the next 20 years avoiding driving until finally deciding to overcome his or her fear.

In cases where an individual is fearful of driving and also lacks basic driving skills, it can be useful to combine exposure practices with driving lessons. Some driving instructors even specialize in training fearful drivers. Such an instructor can be especially helpful because he or she is more likely to be supportive and understanding around the fear, in addition to being able to help the individual to become a better driver.

Social and Communication Skills

Most people with high levels of anxiety in social situations have fine social skills, though they may feel socially awkward from time to time. Furthermore, working on social skills is not necessary for overcoming problems with social anxiety—most people experience a reduction in social anxiety simply through challenging their anxiety-provoking thoughts (Chapter 4) and exposure to feared social situations (Chapters 5 and 6). For some people, though, a lifetime of avoiding social situations may prevent them from mastering some of the subtleties of social interaction. Some of the skills that may be lacking include:

- ✦ Knowing how to ask someone out on a date
- ✦ Basic presentation skills (for example, how to engage an audience during a lecture)
- ✦ Using nonverbal communication and body language effectively (for example, knowing where to stand, posture, eye contact, and the like)
- ✦ How to be assertive
- ✦ Strategies for dealing with disagreements and conflict
- ✦ How to listen to others effectively
- ✦ How to make small talk

Of course, nobody has perfect social skills, and behaviors that work in one situation are not necessarily going to work in others. Being overly focused on having perfect social skills can backfire by increasing your anxiety. Nevertheless, making an effort to improve social skills by making simple changes to one's behavior in social situations may be helpful in some cases.

A full discussion of strategies for improving social skills is beyond the scope of this book, though there are other excellent books on this topic. Furthermore, the website *www.videojug.com* has videos that demonstrate all kinds of social behaviors, including complaining appropriately, looking approachable, making a good first impression, dating, hugging, kissing, and so on. (The site includes video demonstrations of all sorts of nonsocial activities as well, such as how to shave, how to roast a chicken, and how to tie a tie!)

Summary

Most people are able to reduce their anxiety significantly as a result of using the strategies in this book. Nevertheless, challenges do arise from time to time, including difficulty finding the time to practice, difficulty getting motivated, and interference from a variety of other issues, including additional psychological problems, life stresses, medical complications, and a lack of necessary skills. This chapter provides some ideas for how you can deal with these challenges if they seem to be affecting your ability to benefit from the techniques in this book.

13

Living without Anxiety

Y ou should read this chapter once you have tamed your anxiety problem. It will help you develop the skills to keep your anxiety problem away as you shift from *fighting against it* toward *living without it*.

Where Is Your Anxiety Now?

At the beginning of this book, you spent a fair amount of time examining your anxiety and rating how much it affected you and your life. Now that your anxiety has improved, you should go through those steps again, for two reasons:

1. **Seeing how much you have improved can motivate you to maintain those gains.** Few things are as powerful as previous success for increasing your motivation to keep up your hard work. When you see how far you've come, you'll want to protect those improvements and do whatever you can to prevent a return of your anxiety.

2. **Reassessing your anxiety can help you identify areas that are still causing difficulty.** On occasion, when people have made great gains in overcoming their anxiety in most areas of their life, they focus on those improvements while ignoring areas that still cause problems. This can lead to difficulties later because the more leftover symptoms you have now, the more likely the anxiety can creep back and start to take over your life again.

In Chapter 2, you described several aspects of your anxiety and rated how severe they were. Flip back to that chapter and remind yourself of what you wrote. Then copy what you wrote in Chapter 2 in Forms 13.1–13.4.

form 13.1	**Situational Triggers for My Anxiety Problems** (see page 39)	
Anxiety problem	**Situational triggers**	**Does it still trigger my anxiety?**
1.		Yes/No
		Yes/No
		Yes/No
		Yes/No
		Yes/No
		Yes/No
2.		Yes/No
		Yes/No
		Yes/No
		Yes/No
		Yes/No
		Yes/No
3.		Yes/No
		Yes/No
		Yes/No
		Yes/No
		Yes/No
		Yes/No

form 13.2 **Anxiety-Provoking Thoughts Associated with My Anxiety Problems** (see page 48)		
Anxiety problem	**Anxiety-provoking thoughts**	**Do I still have these thoughts?**
1.		Yes/No
		Yes/No
		Yes/No
		Yes/No
		Yes/No
		Yes/No
2.		Yes/No
		Yes/No
		Yes/No
		Yes/No
		Yes/No
		Yes/No
3.		Yes/No
		Yes/No
		Yes/No
		Yes/No
		Yes/No
		Yes/No

form 13.3 **Situations I Avoid** (see page 49)

Anxiety problem	Situations and objects I avoid	Frequency of avoidance from Chap. 2 (0–100)	Frequency of avoidance now (0–100)
1.			
2.			
3.			

form 13.4	**My Safety Behaviors** (see page 53)	
Anxiety problem	**Safety behaviors**	**Do I still use these safety behaviors?**
1.		Yes/No
		Yes/No
		Yes/No
		Yes/No
		Yes/No
		Yes/No
2.		Yes/No
		Yes/No
		Yes/No
		Yes/No
		Yes/No
		Yes/No
3.		Yes/No
		Yes/No
		Yes/No
		Yes/No
		Yes/No
		Yes/No

Look over these lists and compare how you felt when you started this workbook to how you feel now. Have you made the gains you had hoped to? Are you able to do things you couldn't do before? Have you been able to control and change your anxious thinking? Were you able to give up your safety behaviors and face your anxiety head on? For every achievement you've made, you should congratulate yourself. It required hard work, courage, and determination. Congratulations!

You deserve a reward or celebration. Go out for dinner and a movie. Or stay in and cook a nice dinner and rent a movie. Go dancing. Send your kids to their grandparents' house for the night.

While patting yourself on the back for the gains you've made, you might also feel that you still have some goals you haven't reached. Are there areas where you feel you need to keep working? If so, go back to Chapter 4 to review how you can use thought challenging to confront those remaining anxious thoughts, and Chapters 5 through 8 to prepare yourself to confront the situations, thoughts, or physical sensations that continue to provoke your anxiety. Don't worry; this chapter will still be here once you get the remainder of your anxiety problems under control.

I'm Happy with My Improvement—What Now?

If you genuinely feel that you have your anxiety problems under control, then now is the time to shift from *making your gains* to *maintaining your gains.* This doesn't mean closing this book and never thinking about your anxiety again. Even if you feel that you're "cured," anxiety problems can be sneaky and find their way back into your life. Even world-class pianists need to practice their scales every now and then. Similarly, you must practice your anti-anxiety skills periodically to maintain your gains.

A first step is to review which strategies had the biggest impact on your anxiety. For most people, that would be the exposure exercises. Others find greater success with the thought-challenging or relaxation skills. Write down those skills that you feel were most important in your recovery:

1. _____

2. _____

3. _____

Now start to develop a plan to work these strategies into your regular routine. We strongly encourage you to continue practicing these skills. You probably don't need to spend as much time practicing as you did while working through the earlier chapters, but please don't stop! As with anything you've worked to master, you'll lose the skill if you don't keep it alive.

Keeping Up Your Anti-Anxiety Skills

Jamal was a former patient who went through this program because of his intense fears of public speaking and social interactions. He had even refused a promotion at work (and a substantial pay raise) because he was terrified of having to make occasional presentations to the board and to manage the people working under him. During his treatment, he practiced communicating assertively and confidently with his coworkers. He also practiced talking to small audiences.

As he continued his treatment, Jamal started to practice giving presentations to larger and larger audiences. By the time he was finished, he felt very little anxiety when standing up and talking in front of others. He was able to accept the promotion and found that he was more than capable of presenting to the board and managing his department.

But Jamal was wise enough to realize that he needed to continue to work on his anti-anxiety skills. After finishing the program, he joined a local chapter of Toastmasters International. We mentioned this helpful organization earlier. For a small fee, members get together regularly to give talks, presentations, and speeches to improve their speaking skills. Jamal decided to attend these meetings once a month to help him stay on top of his improvements. He also joined the board of his homeowners' association so that he would have opportunities to practice being assertive. Both of these activities were a great help to him in maintaining his improvements.

What about you? What are some activities you could do every now and then to keep your anti-anxiety skills fresh? You don't need to do them daily or even weekly. Here are some examples:

Former Fears	Current Activities
Certain animals	About once a month, go to the zoo, humane society, or other places where you're likely to see your previously feared animal.
Bodily sensations	Every 2 weeks, practice the interoceptive exposure exercises that you found most helpful in Chapter 8.
Social fears	Join groups where you can interact with people. Ask your boss for an opportunity to present at meetings occasionally.
Contamination fears	Each month, for one afternoon, make a point of going out and touching things that used to concern you.
Worries about your family's safety	Every few weeks, pick a day that is going to be your "no cellular phone" day. Go out for the day and practice keeping your worries at bay.

Now, think of what you could do to maintain your gains. Write these ideas down on Form 13.5 and post this list somewhere you will see it and be reminded to keep up your practice.

Predicting and Recovering from Lapses and Relapses

Now for the inevitable reminder: setbacks happen. Many, if not most, people going through this program will have a lapse at some point in the first year or two, especially during times of stress.

But a *lapse* isn't the same as a *relapse*. A *lapse* is a temporary setback in which you experience a return of symptoms or you stop using the skills you learned. You may find yourself avoiding something you should be doing, cleaning something that doesn't really need cleaning, having a panic attack after several panic-free months, triple-checking something when you should trust yourself, worrying excessively about something minor, and so on. Lapses can happen after a bad experience—after a person who used to fear flying has a bumpy flight or a person who had contamination fears comes down with the flu—or they can happen for no obvious reason.

A *relapse*, on the other hand, is a more severe setback, in which your anxiety returns with full force, taking control over some part of your life again. A setback is a relapse if you find yourself back at square one again.

Dealing with Lapses

If you experience a lapse, try not to get worked up over it. It happens to most people. You have the skills to get yourself back on track. Do some thought challenging of the anxious thoughts you're having. Perform your own exposures to get your fears back under control.

The funny thing about lapses is that, in hindsight, you probably could have seen them coming. Lapses usually happen when we're under stress or in a difficult situation. For some, going back to classes after the summer break is a time when they're prone to lapses. Others find that even pleasant times, such as the holiday season or preparing for a vacation, can put them at risk of a lapse.

What about you? Are there times when you feel you might be at greater risk of a lapse or setback? Think about it and make a list.

_____

_____

_____

_____

_____

Strategies for Maintaining Gains

My former fears	My activities for keeping the anxiety away for good
Fear 1	
Fear 2	
Fear 3	

If you know there are times when you might be prone to a lapse, you can prepare yourself in advance. Perhaps you can open up Chapter 9 and practice relaxation exercises. Maybe you can increase how often you practice those skills you decided you would use to maintain your gains. Maybe you can prepare for stressful situations, so they're a little less stressful. Take some time to generate some ideas you can use to prepare for situations where you're at risk for a lapse and then write them down:

_____

_____

_____

_____

Dealing with Relapses

As much as we hope they won't, relapses sometimes happen. Sometimes lapses build up unexpectedly and you find yourself returning to your old anxious patterns. This can feel very discouraging. People often "beat themselves up" for letting that happen.

Rather than punishing yourself for a relapse, take control and remind yourself that you beat the anxiety once before—you can do it again! This time it will be even easier to gain control over your anxiety because you already know what to do. Go back through this program and work through the exercises that helped you previously. Challenge your anxious thoughts and expose yourself to your anxiety triggers again. Resume your relaxation exercises, if these were helpful previously. Look at your lifestyle habits to see if there are areas you can improve. By resuming the strategies that were helpful before, you will regain your control over your anxiety.

What are some signs that you might be having a relapse instead of simply a lapse? Janet previously had agoraphobia, and didn't leave her home for fear that she might have a panic attack. She worked through this program and overcame her fears. She now goes out to malls and crowded places with very little anxiety. But she knows that old habits sometimes have a way of coming back, so she identified several warning signs to alert herself that she might be starting a relapse. She then developed a plan to get back in control of her anxiety (see Form 13.6).

What are your own signs that you might be starting a relapse? Write them down on Form 13.7 and develop your own plan for regaining control. Keep this sheet handy so that at the first sign of trouble, you will know what you need to do.

Moving On

Though it's important to understand that setbacks can happen and to prepare yourself to cope with possible triggers for relapse, focus on what's most important: *the improvements you have made in overcoming your anxiety and taking back your life.*

form 13.6	Janet's Plan for Dealing with Relapses	
Signs of relapse	**My action plan to get back my control**	
I go four straight days without leaving the house.	Immediately pull out this book and challenge my anxious thoughts.
	Get dressed and go to the mall right away to practice my exposures. Do this every day for a week.
I start freaking out about funny sensations in my body.	Immediately pull out this book and challenge my anxious thoughts that something might be wrong with me.
	Reread Chapter 8 and start practicing the exposures to bodily sensations twice a day for 2 weeks.

form 13.7	My Plan for Dealing with Relapses	
Signs of a relapse	**My action plan to get back my control**	

Using the space below, you need to do one more exercise—and then you'll be done with all the forms in this program! First, write down the most important things that you can do now that you couldn't do before because of your anxiety.

1. _____

_____

2. _____

_____

3. _____

_____

4. _____

_____

5. _____

_____

Doesn't it feel spectacular to be able to do these things again (or for the first time)?

Now, write down at least three things that you are *going* to do in the near future that you were prevented from doing because of your anxiety. Maybe take that vacation you avoided because of your fears of flying or driving. Or make the big purchase you put off because of unrealistic financial worries. It even could involve signing up for a dating or singles club now that you've overcome your social fears. What do you want to achieve now that you can?

1. _____

_____

2. _____

_____

3. _____

_____

4. _____

_____

5. _____

_____

Now pick one, and go ahead and do it. You've earned it!

14

A Guide for Family and Friends

From the time we are born to the time we die, we depend on our relationships with others for just about everything: food, shelter, work, education, health care, entertainment, companionship—you name it. In our closest relationships, we have an important effect on each other's emotional lives. The positive emotions we feel sustain us and make life worth living. The negative emotions we feel, such as anxiety, depression, and anger, are often tied to what's happening in our relationships.

If you're close to someone who suffers from anxiety, you're well aware that the anxiety problem affects you too. You may be less aware, though, of how your behavior affects the person's anxiety and of what you can do to help this important person in your life. This chapter is written specifically for the family member, close friend, partner, or other significant presence in the life of someone with anxiety problems. Of course, people who experience anxiety should also read this chapter to learn how their family and friends can be most helpful.

In this chapter, we'll explore issues related to the effects of anxiety on family and friends, as well as your effects on the individual's anxiety. And we'll offer suggestions for ways you can help your loved one with his or her anxiety problem.

The Effect of Anxiety on Family and Friends

How an individual's anxiety affects his or her close circle can vary enormously. Some people hide their anxiety problems completely from their closest friends and family members—even their spouses. In these cases, anxiety would have very little impact on friends and family. At the other extreme, some family members' entire lives seem to revolve around their loved one's anxiety problem. Most of the time, the impact of an individual's anxiety falls somewhere between these extremes.

Dealing with an anxiety disorder in someone you love can be a great source of stress. How many of these stressors do you experience?

✦ **Empathizing with a loved one who is suffering.** Nobody likes to see their loved ones suffer. Having a loved one with an anxiety disorder can be emotionally painful.

✦ **Financial stress.** There is often a relationship between the severity of an anxiety disorder and an individual's earning potential, so family members may have to help out financially because of lost wages (from missed work, turned-down promotions, missed opportunities, and so on). And there may be other financial costs associated with having an anxiety problem (for example, the cost of treatment) that family members have to help cover.

✦ **Conflict in relationships.** Like anxiety, anger is often a response to feeling vulnerable in the face of a perceived threat. Recent research from our clinic and elsewhere has found that many people with anxiety problems report greater than average levels of anger and irritability. Increased irritability can take its toll on anxiety sufferers' loved ones, and can lead to conflict and arguments.

✦ **Helping out with avoided activities.** Depending on the focus of your loved one's anxiety, he or she may be unable to do certain everyday things, such as shopping, driving, traveling, or being home alone. So you may have to do more shopping and driving, or miss out on vacations, or spend more time at home than you would like.

✦ **Helping the individual to feel safe.** You may often be called upon to do things to help the anxiety sufferer feel safe: driving only at particular times or in certain lanes, washing frequently to keep contamination out of the house, checking outside the house for birds or dogs, or phoning frequently to let the anxiety sufferer know that you're safe. These sorts of behaviors can be very time-consuming and stressful for you.

Do you recognize yourself in some of these descriptions? Record all the ways you can think of in which your loved one's anxiety affects you.

_____

_____

_____

_____

_____

_____

_____

How Your Behaviors Affect the Anxiety

Now let's consider what effects you may be having on the person that aren't helpful. Two categories of behavior in particular have been found to have a negative impact on anxiety.

Expressed Emotion

Expressed emotion refers to the ways family members (typically parents or spouses) communicate emotionally toward an individual. Two types of expressed emotion—critical comments and emotional overinvolvement—have been shown to have a negative impact on anxiety. Expressed emotion is assessed by a family interview conducted by a trained professional and resulting in a numerical score. The higher the score, the more unhealthy the family environment is, with the result of increased severity, higher relapse rates, and poorer response to treatment for a wide range of psychological problems (including anxiety problems, schizophrenia, bipolar disorder, and others). High expressed emotion among family members probably doesn't *cause* these problems, but it does tend to make them more severe and more resistant to treatment.

So what are these things you might be doing that are only making the person's anxiety more entrenched? *Critical comments* are statements of dislike, resentment, or annoyance. Communication can be critical based on its content, its tone, or both. It's understandable that you may feel annoyed and resentful at times, but try not to let those feelings out in unconstructive comments. Examples of critical comments to avoid include:

+ "You should be able to pull yourself up by your bootstraps and get yourself to work like everyone else in the family."
+ "You're faking your OCD symptoms to get attention from the rest of us."
+ "If you would stop being so anxious all the time, the rest of the family would probably get along much better."
+ "You're such an idiot! Why can't you just be normal?"

These statements may sound extreme, but perhaps you have made statements like these in milder forms. Can you think of any comments you have made recently that might be perceived as critical? Record examples in the space below. We're not trying to make you feel bad! Only to bring these thoughts to your attention for now.

_____

_____

_____

_____

_____

The other type of expressed emotion that reflects an unhealthy family environment is one in which family members are *emotionally overinvolved* in a person's anxiety problems: overprotective, overly concerned, overly self-sacrificing, or overly blaming of themselves for their loved one's problems. Examples of statements reflecting emotional overinvolvement include:

+ "Your anxiety is causing me so much stress that I think I may have a nervous breakdown."
+ "If you don't get help for your anxiety problem, I'm going to have to quit my job to take care of you."
+ "Your anxiety is all my fault. If I had just been a better parent, this never would have happened."

Do you think others would describe you as emotionally overinvolved with your anxious loved one's problems? Can you think of examples of ways in which you might be? If so, record these examples in the space below.

_____

_____

_____

_____

_____

Family Accommodation

Sometimes, in an effort to be supportive, you might wind up doing things that only make it easier for your loved one to engage in his or her anxious behaviors. This is referred to as *family accommodation*. Some examples would be:

+ Buying extra soap so the person with obsessive–compulsive disorder (OCD) can wash many times per day
+ Allowing a child to stay home from school because of anxiety
+ Doing all the driving for the family, so the person who fears driving doesn't have to do it
+ Working two jobs to support an adult child who has avoided finding work because of a fear of job interviews
+ Checking outside the house for dogs each morning so the person with a fear of dogs can find out if the coast is clear before leaving the house for work
+ Providing constant reassurance to someone with health anxiety who asks everyone (often many times per day) whether the spots on his skin are signs of possible cancer
+ Encouraging someone with extreme social anxiety to have a few drinks before going to a party or to avoid going to the party altogether
+ Going to the shopping mall with a family member who is afraid to go shopping alone
+ Phoning an anxious family member many times each day to make sure that he or she is not worrying about your safety

These all seem like nice things to do to help the person feel less anxious. The problem is that these sorts of behaviors aren't doing anything to help the person overcome his or her anxiety issues.

Most people who live with someone who has an anxiety problem engage in accommodation from time to time. Can you think of ways in which you accommodate your loved one's anxiety? If so, record your examples in the spaces below.

_____

_____

_____

_____

Changing Unhelpful Family Behaviors

There are a number of important do's and don'ts that would be good for you to know so you can help your loved one who suffers from anxiety.

Learn about Your Loved One's Anxiety Problem and Its Treatment

We all know what it feels like to be anxious, afraid, or worried from time to time. Yet those of us who don't have an anxiety disorder may find it very hard to understand how someone can come to develop a full-blown anxiety problem, and we often have misconceptions about anxiety. Below are some examples of the beliefs that people sometimes hold about the anxiety problems experienced by people they care about:

+ "With a bit more willpower, you'd be able to control your anxiety."
+ "Anxiety problems can't be treated."
+ "Anxiety problems should be kept private; nobody outside the family should be allowed to find out about them."
+ "Your anxiety is my fault."
+ "You're crazy."
+ "All your difficult behaviors stem from your anxiety."
+ "You're trying to manipulate me by pretending to be anxious."
+ "Your anxiety will keep getting worse until you're completely unable to function."
+ "I need to do everything I can to make sure you're calm and happy."
+ "It would be terrible if you were to have a panic attack."
+ "If I keep nagging you to do things, it will eventually work."

Though a few of these statements may be true in rare cases, for the most part these are false beliefs. In fact, they reflect a lack of understanding about the nature and treatment of anxiety disorders. Regardless of whether you hold these particular beliefs, chances are you don't fully understand what your loved one is experiencing. One thing you could do to remedy that is to read this book to learn more about the nature and treatment of his or her anxiety problems.

We also recommend that you invite your loved one to talk to you about his or her anxiety, and that you participate in the discussion in a supportive, nonjudgmental way. Finally, if your spouse or partner is receiving therapy for anxiety, it may be helpful for you to sit in on some (or even all) of the sessions, if your partner and the therapist agree. Even if you don't say much, just being there will help you understand the problem and its treatment, and will be one strong way of showing your partner that you care.

View the Anxiety from Your Loved One's Perspective

One of the best ways of understanding what your loved one is going through is to try to view things from his or her perspective. Showing empathy is an important component of any healthy relationship. We're all good at understanding people who share our values and beliefs, but it can be a challenge to get into someone else's head to understand values and beliefs that are very different from our own. Therefore, someone without an anxiety problem may find it difficult to empathize with someone who suffers from severe anxiety. Even people with anxiety problems may have difficulty understanding others who have different anxiety problems.

Yes, it's hard, but you *can* learn to be more empathic to the anxiety sufferer in your life. First, you need to understand that we all hold irrational thoughts and we all experience negative emotions from time to time. What differs between you and someone with an anxiety problem is the content, triggers, frequency, and severity for these irrational or exaggerated responses. Can you think of times when you responded too strongly to a situation (with fear, sadness, or anger)? In the moment, your concerns probably felt very real. The same is true for your loved one's anxiety. Although you may not share his or her fears, when that fear is triggered, the perception of danger or threat feels very real. Understanding this will allow you to offer helpful support that will surely be appreciated.

Ask Your Loved One How You Can Help

There is no single best way to help someone who is experiencing anxiety. Some people do best when their friends and family members participate in "exposure" practices (for example, someone who fears driving might begin practicing with a spouse or friend in the car before working up to driving alone). Some people find it helpful to talk through an anxiety-provoking situation (here you could help the person to use the cognitive strategies described in Chapter 4 in order to think more realistically about feared situations). Others prefer that family members and friends remind them to complete their forms or stop avoiding situations (careful, though—there's a fine line between "reminding" and "nagging"). Some may simply want someone to listen and provide support. Finally, some people may prefer that their friends and family not get involved at all—if that's the case, it's important to respect their wishes.

We suggest that you ask your loved one how you can best be helpful, and whether he or she would like you to participate in the treatment in any way. You can suggest various ways to help, but in the end it is up to your loved one to decide what's best for him or her. Revisit this question every few weeks during the active part of treatment because the person might have a different idea of how to benefit from your help, depending on the phase of treatment.

Be Supportive Rather Than Critical

As discussed earlier, critical comments from family members never help an anxious person improve. It's very important to communicate in a supportive and positive way, rather than focusing on the negative aspects of your loved one's anxiety. We know it's a cliché, but it really is useful to speak to your loved one in the same ways that you want others to speak to you. If he or she is upset by what you have said, chances are good that you have not communicated in a supportive enough way, even if your intentions were good. Supportive responses should let your loved one know that you're concerned, they should not be critical or blaming, and they should let your loved one know that you are there for him or her. It's usually best not to pressure him or her into confronting feared situations. As we have all experienced, pressure and nagging can lead someone to react in exactly the opposite way to what you had in mind.

Try Not to Be Overly Controlling

It's not your job to solve your loved one's anxiety problem. In fact, constant efforts to eliminate it can just make it worse. As we discussed earlier, emotional overinvolvement by family members can get in the way of a person's treatment. If you're feeling overwhelmed and have a tendency to be overinvolved in your loved one's anxiety, here are some ways to relieve your own stress:

- ✦ Encourage your loved one to seek help (but don't try to be your loved one's therapist!).
- ✦ Find ways to be less involved with your loved one's anxiety. Take more time for yourself, and allow your loved one to take greater responsibility for his or her own problem.
- ✦ Consider getting involved in some activity to reduce your stress level, such as exercise, yoga, mindfulness meditation, relaxation training, or a hobby.
- ✦ Consider getting professional help (for example, cognitive-behavioral therapy or medications) for your own stress and anxiety.
- ✦ Consider getting professional help for issues related to your relationship with your loved one (for example, couple therapy or family therapy).

Stop Accommodating

Although accommodation helps your loved one feel more comfortable in the short term, relying on your accommodating behaviors will only bolster his or her anxiety over the long term. It's important to stop accommodating gradually. For example, if you tend to do all the grocery shopping because your loved one is terrified of being in a crowded supermarket alone, the treatment plan might include going to the supermarket with your loved one and gradually increasing the amount of time he or she is in the supermarket without you. In other words, you don't have to stop all your accommodating behaviors at once. You and your loved one can come up with a schedule or plan for how and when you will decrease these behaviors.

Communicate Effectively

Communication is a complex skill. Some components of communication that are important in relationships include knowing how to listen effectively, learning to make requests assertively (rather than using aggressive or passive communication), making sure that your body language matches what you are saying, sharing your feelings and experiences, and dealing with conflict in a productive way. Are there aspects of your own communication that need to be worked on? If so, you may benefit from checking out some good books on communication. Couple and family therapists are also often trained to help people to communicate more effectively.

Troubleshooting

Here are some suggestions for dealing with several challenges that may arise when you're trying to help a loved one deal with an anxiety problem.

If Your Loved One Refuses to Seek Help

If your loved one refuses to seek help, it may be helpful to find out why. (Chapter 12 discusses some reasons why people may be reluctant.) If the reason is rooted in misinformation (for example, the belief that therapy can't help), then some education may be in order. He or she could read this book, or perhaps agree to attend one therapy session, as long he or she doesn't have to commit to any more than that initially.

In some cases, you may decide that refusing help isn't an option. For example, if you are the parent of a 24-year-old son or daughter who is living under your roof and is housebound, unable to work, and unwilling to seek help, you will need to decide whether seeking help must be a condition of continuing to live in your home.

If Family Members Can't Stop Yelling, Arguing, and Fighting

A family environment where everyone is constantly fighting will make it very difficult for your loved one to overcome his or her anxiety problem. You will all need to learn new ways of communicating with one another. (Family therapy can help in this regard.) In some cases, it may be useful for the person with anxiety to have more time away from his or her family (if this is possible, affordable, and so on).

If Family Members Also Have Anxiety Problems

If you suffer from anxiety too, your own problem may affect how well your loved one does in treatment. For example, if you're trying to help your loved one overcome a fear of dogs and you also fear dogs, you may end up subtly giving the impression that you believe dogs are dangerous. Similarly, if you are shy yourself, you might encourage your shy loved one to come right home after work instead of making an attempt to socialize with coworkers. Anything you can do to help get your own anxiety under control may be helpful to your loved one. Working through this book is a good place to start. You may decide you want to seek professional help too.

If Family Members Feel Threatened by Change

Usually, family members and loved ones are very happy to see their anxious friend, relative, or partner begin to experience less anxiety. At the same time, change—even positive change—can be difficult. For example, a man may start to feel a bit insecure if after 15 years of having his wife around all the time (because she was afraid to leave her home), she suddenly feels comfortable going out with friends and isn't around as much. Parents, spouses, and other family members can start to feel they're no longer needed as their anxious loved ones become able to do more on their own.

If you find that you're feeling a bit insecure as your loved one starts to improve, try some of the strategies in Chapter 4 (on challenging anxious thinking) to deal with your own negative thought patterns. Also, having an open and honest conversation in which you let your loved one know how you are feeling may be useful. In our experience, these feelings usually improve over time.

If Family Members Don't Believe in Seeking Help for Emotional Problems

Sometimes, family members are unsupportive when their loved ones seek help for anxiety problems. They may believe that anxiety is a private matter that should stay in the family, or they may believe that therapy is silly, ineffective, or only for "crazy people." They may feel threatened or even jealous at the idea of their loved one telling a therapist about the intimate details of their life. Finally, some people may worry that treatment will convince their spouse or partner to leave the relationship.

None of these concerns is valid. If you feel reluctant to support your loved one's decision to seek therapy, it's important for you to learn more about what happens in therapy and what the likely outcomes will be. Of course, chances are that if you're reading this chapter, you've already decided to learn more about how anxiety is treated.

We wish you luck and patience as you help family members or friends overcome their anxiety. Your input and support will be invaluable as they take some positive steps toward reclaiming their lives. You may find that your relationship is stronger than ever once they're feeling themselves again with your help.

APPENDIX

Helpful Resources

Associations Based in the United States

Though based in the United States, most of these associations offer details for finding therapists and other resources in the United States and Canada, and several offer information on resources in other countries.

Anxiety Disorders Association of America
8730 Georgia Avenue, Suite 600
Silver Spring, MD 20910
Phone: 1-240-485-1001
Fax: 1-240-485-1035
Website: *www.adaa.org*
+ Annual conference (for professionals and consumers)
+ Consumer memberships and professional memberships
+ Information on support groups in the United States, Canada, South Africa, Mexico, and Australia
+ Names of professionals who treat anxiety disorders in the United States, Canada, and elsewhere

Association for Behavioral and Cognitive Therapies (ABCT)
305 Seventh Avenue, 16th Floor
New York, NY 10001-6008
Phone: 1-212-647-1890
Fax: 1-212-647-1865
Website: *www.abct.org*
+ Professional memberships only, but offers referrals to consumers
+ Find a therapist, *http://abct.org/members/Directory/Find_A_Therapist.cfm*

Academy of Cognitive Therapy (ACT)
260 South Broad Street, 18th Floor
Philadelphia, PA 19102
Phone: 1-267-350-7683
E-mail: *info@academyofct.org*
Website: *www.academyofct.org*
✦ Professional memberships only, but offers referrals for consumers to certified cognitive therapists at *info@academyofct.org*

American Academy of Cognitive and Behavioral Psychology
Attn: E. Thomas Dowd, PhD, ABPP
Department of Psychology
Kent State University
Kent, OH 44242-001
Phone: 1-330-672-7664
Fax: 1-330-672-3786
E-mail: *edowd@kent.edu*
Website: *www.americanacademyofbehavioralpsychology.org*
✦ Professional memberships only, but offers referrals for consumers to board-certified psychologists in cognitive-behavioral psychology at *www.americanacademyofbehavioralpsychology.org/AABP/FellowDirectory.htm*

Freedom from Fear
308 Seaview Avenue
Staten Island, NY 10305
Phone: 1-718-351-1717, ext. 24
Email: *help@freedomfromfear.org*
Website: *www.freedomfromfear.org*
✦ National nonprofit advocacy organization for people with anxiety disorders and depression
✦ Newsletter, blogs, bookstore
✦ Information on support groups and other resources

Obsessive Compulsive Foundation
112 Water Street, Suite 501
Boston, MA 02119
Phone: 617- 973-5801
Fax: 617-973-5803
E-mail: *info@ocfoundation.org*
Website: *www.ocfoundation.org*
✦ Annual conference (for professionals and consumers)
✦ Consumer memberships and professional memberships
✦ Names of professionals who treat OCD in the United States, Canada, and elsewhere
✦ List of intensive treatment programs for OCD in the United States

American Psychological Association
750 First Street, NE
Washington, DC 20002-4242
Phone: 1-800-374-2721
Website: *www.apa.org*
+ Professional memberships only, but offers referrals to consumers
+ Referral line: 1-800-964-2000
+ Find a psychologist (*locator.apa.org/*)

American Psychiatric Association
APA Answer Center
1000 Wilson Boulevard, Suite 1825
Arlington, VA 22209
Phone: 1-888-35-PSYCH (or 1-703-907-7300)
E-mail: *apa@psych.org*
Website: *www.psych.org*
+ Professional memberships only, but offers referrals to consumers
+ Referrals to a psychiatrist at *www.healthyminds.org/locateapsychiatrist.cfm*

Associations Based Outside the United States

Anxiety Disorders Association of Canada
ADAC/ACTA
797 Somerset Street West, Suite 39
Ottawa, Ontario K1R 6R3 Canada
Phone: 1-613-722-0236
Fax: 1-613-722-0374
E-mail: *contactus@anxietycanada.ca*
Website: *www.anxietycanada.ca*
+ Consumer memberships and professional memberships
+ Website provides links to other sites with referral options in Canada

International Association of Cognitive Psychotherapy
Website: *www.the-iacp.com*
+ Professional memberships only, but offers referrals for consumers to cognitive therapists at *www.cognitivetherapyassociation.org/refhome.aspx*

British Association for Behavioural and Cognitive Therapies
Victoria Buildings
9–13 Silver Street
Bury BL9 0EU, United Kingdom
Phone: 0161 797 4484
Fax: 0161 797 2670
E-mail: *babcp@babcp.com*
Website: *www.babcp.com*
✦ Professional memberships only, but website includes a "find a therapist" feature for consumers

Australian Association for Cognitive and Behavioural Therapies
P.O. Box 188
Nedlands, WA 6909
Australia
Website: *www.aacbt.org*
✦ Professional memberships only, but website includes a list of CBT practitioners for consumers (click on the "state branches" link on the left, and then click the link at the bottom of the list).

Internet Resources

Although the information in this section was up to date when this book went to press, web pages come and go, and addresses for Internet resources change frequently. For additional information on Internet resources, we suggest doing a search using key words such as "anxiety," "anxiety disorder," "panic disorder," "social anxiety," "phobia," "obsessive–compulsive disorder," "post-traumatic stress disorder," and so on. Note that although we have screened each of these sites, we have not reviewed them in detail, and cannot take responsibility for the accuracy of the information they contain.

Anxieties.com
www.anxieties.com
✦ A very informative anxiety self-help site run by the Anxiety Disorders Treatment Center (and Dr. Reid Wilson) in Durham, North Carolina

Anxiety Treatment Australia
www.anxietyaustralia.com.au
✦ A website that provides information about treatment options in Australia. The site also includes a comprehensive list of helpful resources, including websites (*www.anxietyaustralia. com.au/useful_resources.shtml*)

Anxiety-Panic.com
www.anxiety-panic.com/default.cfm
✦ A search engine for anxiety-related links

Anxiety Disorders Association of America

www.adaa.org

✦ National association for professionals and consumers with an interest in anxiety disorders

CPA Clinical Practice Guidelines for the Management of Anxiety Disorders

ww1.cpa-apc.org:8080/Publications/CJP/supplements/july2006/anxiety_guidelines_2006.pdf

✦ Downloadable treatment guidelines published in 2006 by the Canadian Psychiatric Association

The Depression Center

www.depressioncenter.net

✦ A web-based self-help treatment program for depression

Internet Mental Health

www.mentalhealth.com

✦ Comprehensive website with information on mental health issues

National Alliance on Mental Illness

nami.org

✦ Provides comprehensive resources on a wide range of mental health issues

National Center for PTSD

www.ncptsd.va.gov

✦ Provides information on PTSD and its treatment

NIMH Anxiety Disorders Brochure

www.nimh.nih.gov/health/publications/anxiety-disorders/nimhanxiety.pdf

✦ Downloadable brochure on anxiety disorders published by the National Institute of Mental Health (published 2007)

The Panic Center

www.paniccenter.net

✦ A web-based, self-help treatment program for panic disorder

Sidran Institute

www.sidran.org

✦ Provides information, education, and advocacy for issues related to traumatic stress

Social Phobia/Social Anxiety Association

www.socialphobia.org

✦ Site for a nonprofit organization focused on social phobia and social anxiety

Social Phobia World

www.socialphobiaworld.com

✦ A place for online forums and chats about social phobia

Recommended Readings and Videos

The list below includes readings on relaxation, acceptance, meditation, couples/relationships/communications.

Panic Disorder with and without Agoraphobia

Self-Help Books

Antony, M. M., & McCabe, R. E. (2004). *10 simple solutions to panic: How to overcome panic attacks, calm physical symptoms, and reclaim your life.* Oakland, CA: New Harbinger.

Barlow, D. H., & Craske, M. G. (2007). *Mastery of your anxiety and panic* (4th ed., workbook). New York: Oxford University Press.

Zuercher-White, E. (1997). *An end to panic: Breakthrough techniques for overcoming panic disorder* (2nd ed.). Oakland, CA: New Harbinger.

Professional Books

Craske, M. G., & Barlow, D. H. (2007). *Mastery of your anxiety and panic* (4th ed., therapist guide). New York: Oxford University Press.

Taylor, S. (2000). *Understanding and treating panic disorder: Cognitive and behavioral approaches.* Chichester, UK: Wiley.

Video Resources

Clark, D. M. (1998). *Cognitive therapy for panic disorder* (DVD) (APA Psychotherapy Videotape Series). Washington, DC: American Psychological Association.

Rapee, R. M. (2006). *Fight or flight?: Overcoming panic and agoraphobia* (DVD). New York: Guilford Press.

Social Anxiety Disorder

Self-Help Books

Antony, M. M. (2004). *10 simple solutions to shyness: How to overcome shyness, social anxiety, and fear of public speaking.* Oakland, CA: New Harbinger.

Antony, M. M., & Swinson, R. P. (2008). *The shyness and social anxiety workbook: Proven, step-by-step techniques for overcoming your fear* (2nd ed.). Oakland, CA: New Harbinger.

Hope, D. A., Heimberg, R. G., Juster, H. R., & Turk, C. L. (2000). *Managing social anxiety.* New York: Oxford University Press.

Stein, M. B., & Walker, J. R. (2002). *Triumph over shyness: Conquering shyness and social anxiety.* New York: McGraw-Hill.

Professional Books

Antony, M. M., & Rowa, K. (2008). *Social anxiety disorder: Psychological approaches to assessment and treatment.* Göttingen, Germany: Hogrefe.

Beidel, D. C., & Turner, S. M. (2007). *Shy children, phobic adults: Nature and treatment of social anxiety disorder* (2nd ed.). Washington, DC: American Psychological Association.

Crozier, W. R., & Alden, L. E. (Eds.). (2005). *The essential handbook of social anxiety for clinicians.* Hoboken, NJ: Wiley.

Heimberg, R. G., & Becker, R. E. (2002). *Cognitive-behavioral group therapy for social phobia: Basic mechanisms and clinical strategies.* New York: Guilford Press.

Hofmann, S., & Otto, M. W. (2008). *Cognitive-behavior therapy of social phobia: Evidence-based and disorder specific treatment techniques.* New York: Routledge.

Hope, D. A., Heimberg, R. G., & Turk, C. L. (2006). *Managing social anxiety: A cognitive behavioral therapy approach* (Therapist guide). New York: Oxford University Press.

Video Resources

Albano, A. M. (2006). *Shyness and social phobia* (DVD). Washington, DC: American Psychological Association.

Rapee, R. M. (2006). *I think they think. . . . Overcoming social phobia* (DVD). New York: Guilford Press.

Obsessive–Compulsive Disorder

Self-Help Books

Foa, E. B., & Wilson, R. (2001). *Stop obsessing!: How to overcome your obsessions and compulsions* (rev. ed.). New York: Bantam Books.

Grayson, J. (2004). *Freedom from obsessive–compulsive disorder: A personalized recovery program for living with uncertainty.* New York: Berkley.

Hyman, B. M., & Pedrick, C. (2005). *The OCD workbook: Your guide to breaking free from obsessive–compulsive disorder* (2nd ed.). Oakland, CA: New Harbinger.

Munford, P. R. (2004). *Overcoming compulsive checking: Free your mind from OCD.* Oakland, CA: New Harbinger.

Munford, P. R. (2005). *Overcoming compulsive washing: Free your mind from OCD.* Oakland, CA: New Harbinger.

Purdon, C., & Clark, D. A. (2005). *Overcoming obsessive thoughts: How to gain control of your OCD.* Oakland, CA: New Harbinger.

Steketee, G., & Frost, R. O. (2007). *Compulsive hoarding and acquiring* (Workbook). New York: Oxford University Press.

Tolin, D., Frost, R. O., & Steketee, G. (2007). *Buried in treasures: Help for compulsive acquiring, saving, and hoarding.* New York: Oxford University Press.

Professional Books

Abramowitz, J. S. (2006). *Obsessive–compulsive disorder.* Cambridge, MA: Hogrefe & Huber.

Abramowitz, J. S. (2006). *Understanding and treating obsessive–compulsive disorder: A cognitive behavioral approach.* Mahwah, NJ: Erlbaum.

Abramowitz, J. S., & Houts, A. C. (Eds.). (2005). *Obsessive–compulsive disorder: Concepts and controversies.* New York: Springer.

Abramowitz, J. S., McKay, D., & Taylor, S. (2008). *Obsessive–compulsive disorder: Subtypes and spectrum conditions.* New York: Elsevier.

Antony, M. M., Purdon, C., & Summerfeldt, L. J. (2007). *Psychological treatment of obsessive–compulsive disorder: Fundamentals and beyond.* Washington, DC: American Psychological Association.

Clark, D. A. (2004). *Cognitive-behavioral therapy for OCD.* New York: Guilford Press.

Rachman, S. (2003). *The treatment of obsessions.* New York: Oxford University Press.

Rachman, S. (2006). *Fear of contamination: Assessment and treatment.* New York: Oxford University Press.

Steketee, G., & Frost, R. O. (2007). *Compulsive hoarding and acquiring* (Therapist guide). New York: Oxford University Press.

Wilhelm, S., & Steketee, G. S. (2006). *Cognitive therapy for obsessive–compulsive disorder: A guide for professionals.* Oakland, CA: New Harbinger.

Video Resources

Antony, M. M. (2007). *Obsessive–compulsive behavior* (DVD). Washington, DC: American Psychological Association.

Wilson, R. R. (2005). *Obsessive–compulsive disorder* (DVD). Washington, DC: American Psychological Association.

OCD "Spectrum" Disorders (Health Anxiety, Trichotillomania, Body Dysmorphic Disorder)

Self-Help Books

Asmundson, G. J. G., & Taylor, S. (2005). *It's not all in your head: How worrying about your health could be making you sick–and what you can do about it.* New York: Guilford Press.

Keuthen, N. J., Stein, D. J., & Christenson, G. A. (2001). *Help for hair pullers: Understanding and coping with trichotillomania.* Oakland, CA: New Harbinger.

Penzel, F. (2003). *The hair pulling problem: A complete guide to trichotillomania.* New York: Oxford University Press.

Wilhelm, S. (2006). *Feeling good about the way you look: A program for overcoming body image problems.* New York: Guilford Press.

Professional Books

Abramowitz, J. S., McKay, D., & Taylor, S. (2008). *Obsessive–compulsive disorder: Subtypes and spectrum conditions.* New York: Elsevier.

Franklin, M. E., & Tolin, D. F. (2007). *Treating trichotillomania: Cognitive-behavioral therapy for hair pulling and related problems.* New York: Springer.

Furer, P., Walker, J. R., & Stein, M. B. (2007). *Treating health anxiety and fear of death: A practitioner's guide.* New York: Springer.

Taylor, S., & Asmundson, G. J. G. (2004). *Treating health anxiety: A cognitive-behavioral approach.* New York: Guilford Press.

Generalized Anxiety Disorder and Chronic Worry

Self-Help Books

Gyoerkoe, K. L., & Wiegartz, P. S. (2006). *10 simple solutions to worry: How to calm your mind, relax your body, and reclaim your life.* Oakland, CA: New Harbinger.

Hazlett-Stevens, H. (2005). *Women who worry too much: How to stop worry and anxiety from ruining relationships, work, and fun.* Oakland, CA: New Harbinger.

Professional Books

Davey, G. C. L., & Wells, A. (Eds.). (2006). *Worry and its psychological disorders: Theory, assessment, and treatment.* Chichester, UK: Wiley.

Dugas, M. J., & Robichaud, M. (2007). *Cognitive-behavioral treatment for generalized anxiety disorder.* New York: Routledge.

Hazlett-Stevens, H. (2008). *Psychological approaches to generalized anxiety disorder: A clinician's guide to assessment and treatment.* New York: Springer.

Heimberg, R. G., Turk, C. L., & Mennin, D. S. (Eds.). (2004). *Generalized anxiety disorder: Advances in research and practice.* New York: Guilford Press.

Rygh, J. L., & Sanderson, W. C. (2004). *Treating generalized anxiety disorder: Evidence-based strategies, tools, and techniques.* New York: Guilford Press.

Specific Phobia

Self-Help Books

Antony, M. M., Craske, M. G., & Barlow, D. H. (2006). *Mastering your fears and phobias* (2nd ed., workbook). New York: Oxford University Press.

Antony, M. M., & McCabe, R. E. (2005). *Overcoming animal and insect phobias: How to conquer fear of dogs, snakes, rodents, bees, spiders, and more.* Oakland, CA: New Harbinger.

Antony, M. M., & Rowa, K. (2007). *Overcoming fear of heights: How to conquer acrophobia and live a life without limits.* Oakland, CA: New Harbinger.

Antony, M. M., & Watling, M. (2006). *Overcoming medical phobias: How to conquer fear of blood, needles, doctors, and dentists.* Oakland, CA: New Harbinger.

Brown, D. (1996). *Flying without fear.* Oakland, CA: New Harbinger.

Triffitt, J. (2003). *Back in the driver's seat: Understanding, challenging, and managing fear of driving.* Tasmania, Australia: Dr. Jacqui Triffitt (*www.backinthedriversseat.com.au*).

Professional Books

Craske, M. G., Antony, M. M., & Barlow, D. H. (2006). *Mastering your fears and phobias* (2nd ed., therapist guide). New York: Oxford University Press.

Maj, M., Akiskal, H. S., López-Ibor, J. J., & Okasha, A. (2004). *Phobias.* Hoboken, NJ: Wiley.

Trauma and Posttraumatic Stress Disorder

Self-Help Books

Follette, V. M., & Pistorello, J. (2007). *Finding life beyond trauma: Using acceptance and commitment therapy to heal from post-traumatic stress and trauma-related problems.* Oakland, CA: New Harbinger.

Hickling, E. J., & Blanchard, E. B. (2006). *Overcoming the trauma of your motor vehicle accident: A cognitive-behavioral treatment program* (Workbook). New York: Oxford University Press.

Rothbaum, B. O., Foa, E. B., & Hembree, E. A. (2007). *Reclaiming your life from a traumatic experience* (Workbook). New York: Oxford University Press.

Professional Books

Foa, E. B., Hembree, E. A., & Rothbaum, B. O. (2007). *Prolonged exposure therapy for PTSD: Emotional processing of traumatic experiences* (Therapist guide). New York: Oxford University Press.

Foa, E. B., & Rothbaum, B. O. (1998). *Treating the trauma of rape: Cognitive behavioral therapy for PTSD.* New York: Guilford Press.

Hickling, E. J., & Blanchard, E. B. (2006). *Overcoming the trauma of your motor vehicle accident: A cognitive-behavioral treatment program* (Therapist guide). New York: Oxford University Press.

Resick, P. A., & Schnicke, M. K. (1996). *Cognitive processing therapy for rape victims: A treatment manual.* Newbury Park, CA: Sage.

Taylor, S. (2006). *Clinician's guide to PTSD: A cognitive-behavioral approach.* New York: Guilford Press.

Wilson, J. P., & Keane, T. M. (Eds.). (2004). *Assessing psychological trauma and PTSD* (2nd ed.). New York: Guilford Press.

Zayfert, C., & Becker, C. B. (2007). *Cognitive-behavioral therapy for PTSD: A case formulation approach.* New York: Guilford Press.

Anxiety Disorders in Children and Adolescents

Self-Help Books

Crist, J. J. (2004). *What to do when you're scared and worried: A guide for kids.* Minneapolis, MN: Free Spirit.

Eisen, A. R., & Engler, L. B. (2006). *Helping your child with separation anxiety: A step-by-step guide for parents.* Oakland, CA: New Harbinger.

Fitzgibbons, L., & Pedrick, C. (2003). *Helping your child with OCD.* Oakland, CA: New Harbinger.

Foa, E. B., & Andrews, L. W. (2006). *If your adolescent has an anxiety disorder: An essential resource for parents.* New York: Oxford University Press.

Kearney, C. A., & Albano, A. M. (2007). *When children refuse school: A cognitive behavioral therapy approach* (Parent workbook). New York: Oxford University Press.

Last, C. G. (2006). *Help for worried kids: How your child can conquer anxiety and fear.* New York: Guilford Press.

McHolm, A. E., Cunningham, C. E., & Vanier, M. K. (2005). *Helping your child with selective mutism: Practical steps to overcome a fear of speaking.* Oakland, CA: New Harbinger.

Piacentini, J., Langley, A., & Roblek, T. (2007). *It's only a false alarm* (Workbook). New York: Oxford University Press.

Rapee, R. M., Spence, S. H., Cobham, V., & Wignall, A. (2000). *Helping your anxious child: A step-by-step guide for parents.* Oakland, CA: New Harbinger.

Wagner, A. P. (2000). *Up and down the worry hill.* Rochester, NY: Lighthouse Press.

Wagner, A. P. (2002). *What to do when your child had obsessive–compulsive disorder: Strategies and solutions.* Rochester, NY: Lighthouse Press.

Wagner, A. P. (2002). *Worried no more: Help and hope for anxious children.* Rochester, NY: Lighthouse Press.

Professional Books

Albano, A. M., & DiBartolo, P. M. (2007). *Cognitive-behavioral therapy for social phobia in adolescents: Stand up, speak out.* New York: Oxford University Press.

Chorpita, B. F. (2007). *Modular cognitive-behavioral therapy for childhood anxiety disorders.* New York: Guilford Press.

Kearney, C. A. (2005). *Social anxiety and social phobia in youth: Characteristics, assessment, and psychological treatment.* New York: Springer.

Kearney, C. A., & Albano, A. M. (2007). *When children refuse school: A cognitive-behavioral therapy approach* (2nd ed., therapist guide). New York: Oxford University Press.

March, J. S., & Mulle, K. (1998). *OCD in children and adolescents.* New York: Guilford Press.

Mattick, S. G., & Ollendick, T. H. (2002). *Panic disorder and anxiety in adolescents.* Malden, MA: Blackwell.

Morris, T. L., & March, J. S. (Eds.). (2004). *Anxiety disorders in children and adolescents* (2nd ed.). New York: Guilford Press.

Ollendick, T. H., & March, J. S. (Eds.). (2004). *Phobic and anxiety disorders in children and adolescents: A clinician's guide to effective psychosocial and pharmacological interventions.* New York: Oxford University Press.

Piacentini, J., Langley, A., & Roblek, T. (2007). *Cognitive-behavioral treatment of childhood OCD: It's only a false alarm* (Therapist guide). New York: Oxford University Press.

Rapee, R. M., Wignall, A., Hudson, J. L., & Schniering, C. A. (2000). *Treating anxious children and adolescents: An evidence-based approach.* Oakland, CA: New Harbinger.

Anxiety Disorders and Related Topics (General)

Self-Help Books

Antony, M. M., & Swinson, R. P. (2008). *When perfect isn't good enough: Strategies for coping with perfectionism* (2nd ed.). Oakland, CA: New Harbinger.

Bourne, E. J. (2003). *Coping with anxiety: 10 simple ways to relieve anxiety, fear and worry.* Oakland, CA: New Harbinger.

Bourne, E. J. (2005). *The anxiety and phobia workbook* (4th ed.). Oakland, CA: New Harbinger.

Professional Books

Antony, M. M., Orsillo, S. M., & Roemer, L. (Eds.). (2001). *Practitioner's guide to empirically based measures of anxiety.* New York: Springer.

Antony, M. M., & Stein, M. B. (2009). *Oxford handbook of anxiety and related disorders.* New York: Oxford University Press.

Antony, M. M., & Swinson, R. P. (2000). *Phobic disorders and panic in adults: A guide to assessment and treatment.* Washington, DC: American Psychological Association.

Barlow, D. H. (2002). *Anxiety and its disorders: The nature and treatment of anxiety and panic* (2nd ed.). New York: Guilford Press.

Beck, A. T., & Emery, G. (1985). *Anxiety disorders and phobias: A cognitive perspective.* New York: Basic Books.

Dozois, D. J. A., & Dobson, K. S. (2004). *The prevention of anxiety and depression: Theory, research, and practice.* Washington, DC: American Psychological Association.

Kase, L., & Ledley, D. (2007). *Anxiety disorders.* Hoboken, NJ: Wiley.

Nutt, D. J., & Ballenger, J. C. (2003). *Anxiety disorders.* Malden, MA: Blackwell Science.

Rosqvist, J. (2005). *Exposure treatments for anxiety disorders: A practitioner's guide to concepts, methods, and evidence-based practice.* New York: Brunner-Routledge.

Medication Treatments

Bezchlibnyk-Butler, K. Z., Jeffries, J. J., & Virani, A. S. (2007). *Clinical handbook of psychotropic drugs* (17th ed.). Ashland, OH: Hogrefe.

Canadian Pharmacists Association. (2008). *Compendium of pharmaceuticals and specialties: The Canadian drug reference for professionals.* Ottawa, ON: Author.

Physicians' desk reference (62nd ed.). (2008). Montvale, NJ: Thomson PDR.

Swinson, R. P., Antony, M. M., Bleau, P., Chokka, P., Craven, M., Fallu, A., et al. (2006). Clinical practice guidelines: Management of anxiety disorders. *Canadian Journal of Psychiatry, 51*(suppl. 2), 1S–92S.

Communication Skills and Couples Issues

Self-Help Books

Berry, D. M. (2005). *Romancing the web: A therapist's guide to the finer points of online dating.* Manitowoc, WI: Blue Water.

Bolton, R. (1979). *People skills.* New York: Simon & Schuster.

Christensen, A., & Jacobson, N. S. (2000). *Reconcilable differences.* New York: Guilford Press.

Davis, M., Paleg, K., & Fanning, P. (2004). *The messages workbook: Powerful strategies for effective communication at work and home.* Oakland, CA: New Harbinger.

Honeychurch, C., & Watrous, A. (2003). *Talk to me: Conversation tips for the small-talk challenged.* Oakland, CA: New Harbinger.

Jacobson, B., & Gordon, S. J. (2004). *The shy single: A bold guide to dating for the less-than-bold dater.* Emmaus, PA: Rodale.

Katz, E. M. (2003). *I can't believe I'm buying this book: A commonsense guide to successful Internet dating.* Berkeley, CA: 10 Speed Press.

MacInnis, J. L. (2006). *The elements of great public speaking: How to be calm, confident, and compelling.* Berkeley, CA: 10 Speed Press.

McKay, M., Davis, M., & Fanning, P. (1995). *Messages: The communications skills book* (2nd ed.). Oakland, CA: New Harbinger.

McKay, M., Fanning, P., & Paleg, K. (2006). *Couple skills: Making your relationship work* (2nd ed.). Oakland, CA: New Harbinger.

Monarth, H., & Kase, L. (2007). *The confident speaker: Beat your nerves and communicate at your best in any situation.* New York: McGraw-Hill.

Patterson, R. J. (2000). *The assertiveness workbook: How to express your ideas and stand up for yourself at work and in relationships.* Oakland, CA: New Harbinger.

Stein, M. (2003). *Fearless interviewing: How to win the job by communicating with confidence.* New York: McGraw-Hill.

Mindfulness-, Relaxation-, and Acceptance-Based Approaches

Self-Help Books

Davis, M., Eshelman, E. R., & McKay, M. (2008). *The relaxation and stress reduction workbook* (6th ed.). Oakland, CA: New Harbinger.

Forsyth, J. P., & Eifert, G. H. (2007). *The mindfulness and acceptance workbook for anxiety: A guide to breaking free from anxiety, phobias, and worry using acceptance and commitment therapy.* Oakland, CA: New Harbinger.

Kabat-Zinn, J. (1990). *Full catastrophe living: Using the wisdom of your body and mind to face stress, pain, and illness.* New York: Dell.

Professional Books

Bernstein, D. A., Borkovec, T. D., & Hazlett-Stevens, H. (2000). *New directions in progressive relaxation training: A guidebook for helping professionals.* Westport, CT: Praeger.

Eifert, G. H., & Forsyth, J. P. (2005). *Acceptance and commitment therapy for anxiety disorders: A practitioner's treatment guide to using mindfulness, acceptance, and values-based behavior change strategies.* Oakland, CA: New Harbinger.

Hayes, S. C., Strosahl, K. D., & Wilson, K. G. (1999). *Acceptance and commitment therapy: An experiential approach to behavior change.* New York: Guilford Press.

Orsillo, S. M., & Roemer, L. (Eds.). (2005). *Acceptance- and mindfulness-based approaches to anxiety: Conceptualization and treatment.* New York: Springer.

Cognitive and Behavioral Therapy (General)

Self-Help Books

Burns, D. D. (1999). *The feeling good handbook* (rev. ed.). New York: Plume.

Butler, G., & Hope, T. (2007). *Managing your mind: The mental fitness guide* (2nd ed.). New York: Oxford University Press.

Goudey, P. (2000). *The unofficial guide to beating stress.* New York: IDG Books.

Greenberger, D., & Padesky, C. A. (1995). *Mind over mood: Change how you feel by changing the way you think.* New York: Guilford Press.

McKay, M., Davis, M., & Fanning, P. (2007). *Thoughts and feelings: Taking control of your moods and your life* (3rd ed.). Oakland, CA: New Harbinger.

Professional Books

Antony, M. M., & Barlow, D. H. (Eds.). (2002). *Handbook of assessment and treatment planning for psychological disorders.* New York: Guilford Press.

Antony, M. M., Ledley, D. R., & Heimberg, R. G. (Eds.). (2005). *Improving outcomes and preventing relapse in cognitive-behavioral therapy.* New York: Guilford Press.

Arkowitz, H., Westra, H. A., Miller, W. R., & Rollnick, S. (Eds.). (2008). *Motivational interviewing in the treatment of psychological problems.* New York: Guilford Press.

Barlow, D. H. (Ed.) (2008). *Clinical handbook of psychological disorders* (4th ed.): A step-by-step treatment manual. New York: Guilford Press.

Beck, J. S. (1995). *Cognitive therapy: Basics and beyond.* New York: Guilford Press.

Beck, J. S. (2005). *Cognitive therapy for challenging problems: What to do when the basics don't work.* New York: Guilford Press.

Bieling, P. J., McCabe, R. E., & Antony, M. M. (2006). *Cognitive-behavioral therapy in groups.* New York: Guilford Press.

Friedberg, R. D., & McClure, J. M. (2002). *Clinical practice of cognitive therapy with children and adolescents: The nuts and bolts.* New York: Guilford Press.

Leahy, R. L. (2003). *Cognitive therapy techniques: A practitioner's guide.* New York: Guilford Press.

Miller, W. R., & Rollnick, S. (2002). *Motivational interviewing: Preparing people for change* (2nd ed.). New York: Guilford Press.

O'Donohue, W., Fisher, J. E., & Hayes, S. C. (Eds.). (2003). *Cognitive behavior therapy: Applying empirically supported techniques in your practice.* Hoboken, NJ: Wiley.

Richard, D. C. S., & Lauterbach, D. (2007). *Handbook of exposure therapies.* New York: Academic Press.

Wright, J. H., Basco, M. R., & Thase, M. E. (2006). *Learning cognitive-behavior therapy: An illustrated guide.* Washington, DC: American Psychiatric Press.

Video Resources

Antony, M. M. (2008). *Cognitive behavioral therapy for perfectionism over time* (DVD). Washington, DC: American Psychological Association.

Beck, J. S. (2006). *Cognitive therapy* (DVD). Washington, DC: American Psychological Association.

Padesky, C. (2008) *Guided discovery using Socratic dialog* (DVD). May be ordered from *www.padesky.com.*

Padesky, C. (2008) *Testing automatic thoughts with thought records* (DVD). May be ordered from *www.padesky.com.*

INDEX

Abdominal discomfort, 14, 154
Abilify (aripiprazole), 187
Acceptance and commitment therapy, 33
Acceptance-based treatments
  choosing among treatment strategies, 74, 76
  developing a treatment plan and, 75
  overview, 33, 169–170
  resources for, 255
Accidents, posttraumatic stress disorder and, 18–19
Accommodation behaviors from family and friends, 237–238, 240–241
Acupuncture, 190
Acute stress disorder, 13
Addiction to medications, 173
Adolescents, resources for, 252–253
Aggressive obsessions, 20. See also Obsessions; Obsessive-compulsive disorder
Agoraphobia
  beliefs often associated with, 30
  identifying safety behaviors you use with, 51
  identifying variables that affect your fear and anxiety and, 40
  identifying your thoughts associated with, 45
  identifying your triggers and, 36
  overview, 13, 15–16
  panic disorder and, 15–16
  resources for, 248
Alcohol use, 176, 203–204, 205–206
Alprazolam, 185
Alternative beliefs, assumptions and predictions, 89
Anger, 9, 80
Animal phobias. See also Specific phobia
  exposure techniques and, 128, 129, 132, 132–133
  identifying safety behaviors you use with, 52
  identifying variables that affect your fear and anxiety and, 40
  identifying your thoughts associated with, 46
  identifying your triggers and, 37
  overview, 18
Anti-anxiety medications, 32, 171–173, 184–186. See also Medication treatments
Anticonvulsants, 186
Antidepressants, 32, 171–173, 178–184. See also Medication treatments
Antipsychotics, 187
Anxiety, thoughts and, 80

Anxiety disorder not otherwise specified (ADNOS), 14, 23
Anxiety disorders
  acute stress disorder, 13
  agoraphobia, 13
  anxiety disorder not otherwise specified (ADNOS), 14, 23
  anxiety due to a general medical condition, 14
  beliefs often associated with, 30
  causes of, 25–31
  in children and adolescents (resource list), 252–253
  description of, 12–23
  distinguishing between, 25
  generalized anxiety disorder, 14, 21–22
  list of, 13–14
  obsessive-compulsive disorder, 13, 19–21
  overview, 34
  panic disorder, 13, 14–16
  posttraumatic stress disorder, 13, 18–19
  resources for, 252–253, 253–254
  separation anxiety disorder, 14, 22
  social anxiety disorder, 13, 16–17
  specific phobia, 13, 17–18
  substance-induced anxiety disorder, 14, 23
  treatments for, 31–33
Anxiety Disorders Association of America (ADAA), 71
Anxiety due to a general medical condition, 14
Anxiety in general
  anxiety vs. fear, 8–9
  causes of, 25–31
  examples of, 1–2
  identifying internal experiences that you fear and avoid, 50, 52, 54
  identifying safety behaviors you use with, 51
  identifying situations and objects that you avoid, 47, 49
  identifying variables that affect, 38, 40–41, 42
  identifying variables that affect your fear and anxiety and, 40
  identifying your physical sensations associated with, 41, 43, 44
  identifying your thoughts associated with, 43, 45, 45–47
  identifying your triggers and, 36
  overview, 1–3, 8–12
  relationship between fear and anxiety, 9

  triggers of anxiety, 10–12
Anxiety Thought Record, 90, 92, 93
Anxiolytics, 32. See also Medication treatments
Appearance preoccupation, 24
Appliances, anxiety concerning, 131
Arranging compulsion, 21. See also Compulsions; Obsessive-compulsive disorder
Assault, posttraumatic stress disorder and, 18–19
Assertiveness, exposure techniques and, 130
Assessment, medication and, 174
Assessment of yourself. See Self-assessment
Association for Behavioral and Cognitive Therapies, 72
Assumptions
  causes of anxiety and, 29, 30
  changing, 86–103
  identifying, 87–88, 103
  overview, 84–85
  problems you may encounter when working with, 103, 105
  relationship between feelings and, 79–80
Ativan (lorazepam), 32. See also Medication treatments
Attention, biased, 81–82
Aurorix (moclobemide), 183–184
Authority figures, fear of, 130
Avoidance
  of bodily sensations, 148–150
  effects of, 148–150, 235
  external triggers and, 11
  identifying internal experiences that you fear and avoid, 50, 52, 54
  identifying situations and objects that you avoid, 47, 49
  overview, 8
  panic disorder and, 15–16
  posttraumatic stress disorder and, 19
  relapse prevention and, 224
  role of, 81–82
Awareness of surroundings, posttraumatic stress disorder and, 19

Behavior, causes of anxiety and, 29, 31
Behavioral approaches to treatment, 32–33, 255–256
Beliefs. See also Core beliefs
  anxiety disorders and, 30
  causes of anxiety and, 29, 30
  changing, 86–103
  core beliefs, 85

Beliefs (*cont.*)
   identifying, 88, 103
   problems you may encounter when
      working with, 103, 105
   relationship between feelings and,
      79–80
Benefits of anxiety, 10
Benzodiazepines, 32, 184–186. *See also*
   Medication treatments
Beta-adrenergic blockers, 186–187
Biased attention, role of, 81–82
Biological causes, 26–27
Biological treatments, 32. *See also*
   Medication treatments
Blink (Gladwell), 81
Blood/injection/injury phobias. *See
   also* Specific phobia
   identifying safety behaviors you use
      with, 52
   identifying variables that affect your
      fear and anxiety and, 40
   identifying your thoughts associated
      with, 46
   identifying your triggers and, 37
   overview, 18
Blurred vision, exposures and, 153
Bodily sensations. *See* Physical
   response
Body dysmorphic disorder
   overview, 24
   resources for, 250
Body-related obsessions, 20. *See also*
   Obsessions; Obsessive-compulsive
   disorder
Brain chemistry as a cause of anxiety,
   26–27
Breathing retraining, 166–168
Breathing symptoms, 14, 152, 153, 154
Buspirone, 186

Caffeine, 202–203, 205–206
Calmness, thoughts and, 80
Catastrophizing (catastrophic
   thinking), 83–84, 95, 98–99
Causes of anxiety and anxiety
   disorders, 25–31
CBT. *See* Cognitive-behavioral therapy
Checking compulsion, 21, 131. *See
   also* Compulsions; Obsessive-
   compulsive disorder
Chest pain/discomfort, 14, 152
Children, resources for anxiety in,
   252–253
Chills, 15, 153
Choking feelings, 14, 152, 154
Cipralex (escitalopram), 179
Claustorphobia. *See* Specific phobia
Cleaning compulsion, 21. *See also*
   Compulsions; Obsessive-
   compulsive disorder
Clomipramine, 182, 183
Clonazepam, 185
Clozaril (clozapine), 187
Cognitive approaches to treatment
   choosing among treatment
      strategies, 73
   developing a treatment plan and, 75
   overview, 32
   resources for, 255–256
   stress management and, 213, 216
Cognitive triggers, 11–12
Cognitive-behavioral therapy, 3, 255–
   256. *See also* Behavioral approaches
   to treatment; Cognitive approaches
   to treatment

Combat, posttraumatic stress disorder
   and, 18–19
Communication skills
   changing unhelpful family behavior
      and, 241
   how behaviors by others affect the
      anxiety and, 236
   overview, 219–220
   resources for, 254
Complementary therapies, 188–190
Compulsions. *See also* Obsessive-
   compulsive disorder; Urges
   anxiety-provoking impulses, 86
   causes of anxiety and, 29, 31
   choosing among treatment
      strategies, 74–75, 76
   identifying internal experiences that
      you fear and avoid, 52, 54–55
   list of, 21
   overview, 19–20
   removing false-safety behaviors and,
      118–123
Confidence, exposure techniques and,
   109
Contamination obsessions, 20, 131.
   See also Obsessions; Obsessive-
   compulsive disorder
Control issues, 24, 340
Core beliefs. *See also* Beliefs
   changing, 101, 103, 104
   identifying, 88
   overview, 85
Cost and benefits of treating your
   anxiety, 60, 61–62, 210
Counselors, seeking help from, 70–
   72
Counting compulsion, 21. *See
   also* Compulsions; Obsessive-
   compulsive disorder
Courage, exposure techniques and,
   109
Crowds, fear of, 130
Cultural causes, 31

Dangers, fear and, 8–9
Dark, fear of. *See* Specific phobia
Death, fear of, 24
Decatastrophizing technique, 95,
   98–99, 169–170
Depression, as an obstacle to treating
   your anxiety, 208–209
Detachment feelings, panic attacks
   and, 15
Diagnosis of anxiety disorders, 12,
   13–14
*Diagnostic and Statistical Manual of
   Mental Disorders* (DSM-IV-TR). *See*
   DSM-IV-TR
Diaphragmatic breathing, 166–168
Diazepam, 185
Diet, 195–197
Direct experience as a cause of anxiety,
   28
Dirt, fear of, 131
Disasters, posttraumatic stress disorder
   and, 18–19
Disorganization, fear of, 131
Dizziness, 15, 33, 152, 153
Doctors, seeking help from, 70–72
Driving, fear of, 219. *See* Specific
   phobia
Drug use, 176, 202–205
DSM-IV-TR (*Diagnostic and Statistical
   Manual of Mental Disorders*), 12
Dying, fear of, 15

Eating disorders, as an obstacle to
   treating your anxiety, 208–209
Edronax (reboxetine), 184
Educating yourself, changing thoughts,
   beliefs, and assumptions with, 92,
   94
Effexor (venlafaxine), 32, 182. *See also*
   Medication treatments
Emotional overinvolvement, 236–237
Enclosed places, fear of. *See* Specific
   phobia
Endorphins, physical exercise and, 200
Environmental phobias, 18. *See also*
   Specific phobia
Escape, external triggers and, 11
Evaluating the evidence technique
   changing core beliefs and, 103
   overview, 89, 92–103, 96–98
Evidence evaluation. *See* Evaluating the
   evidence technique
Exactness and symmetry obsessions,
   20. *See also* Obsessions; Obsessive-
   compulsive disorder
Exercise, physical, 200–202
Experiences as a cause of anxiety,
   28–29
Experiment Form, 100, 101
Experiments technique, 99–100, 101–102
Exposure Plans
   examples of, 128–135
   form for, 110
   overview, 111–117, 123–124
   troubleshooting, 135
Exposure techniques in treatment. *See
   also* Exposures
   acceptance-based treatments and,
      169–170
   choosing among treatment
      strategies, 73–74
   developing a treatment plan and, 75
   Exposure Plans, 110, 111–117,
      123–124, 128–135
   how it works, 108–109
   overview, 32–33, 107, 123–124
   planning the details of, 126–128
   removing false-safety behaviors,
      118–123
   repeating, 117–118
   to thoughts, memories, images and
      urges, 138–147
Exposures. *See also* Exposure
   techniques in treatment
   to animals, 128, 129, 132–133
   to feelings and sensations, 150–154
   to objects and situations, 125–126,
      131–132
   to people, 128, 130, 132–135
   to places, 126–127
   planning the details of, 126–128
   to thoughts, memories, images and
      urges, 138–147
Expressed emotion, 236–237
External triggers, 11
Extrinsic reasons for change, 210–211

Faintness, 15, 152, 153
False-safety behaviors, 118–123,
   203–204. *See also* Safety behaviors
Family
   changing unhelpful behavior from,
      238–241
   effect of anxiety on, 234–235
   how behaviors by affect the anxiety,
      235–238
   troubleshooting, 241–242

Family accommodation, 237–238, 240–241

Family support, 66, 69–70. *See also* Family

Fear
anxiety vs., 8–9
choosing among treatment strategies, 74–75, 76
developing a treatment plan and, 75
exposure techniques and, 108–109
identifying internal experiences that you fear and avoid, 50, 52, 54
identifying situations and objects that you avoid, 47, 49
identifying variables that affect, 38, 40–41, 42
identifying your physical sensations associated with, 41, 43, 44
identifying your thoughts associated with, 43, 45–47
overview, 9–10
panic disorder and, 14–15
relationship of between anxiety and, 9
trauma and, 19
triggers of, 10–12

Fear of losing control, panic attacks and, 15

Fear ratings, exposure techniques and, 115–117

Feelings, physical, 148–150, 148–156. *See also* Physical response

Feelings, relationship between thoughts and, 79–82

"Fight-or-flight" response, 9

Financial challenges
choosing among medications and, 177
as an obstacle to treating your anxiety, 64
overview, 235
seeking professional help and, 71

Flashbacks, 86, 143–144. *See also* Imagery, anxiety-provoking

Flooding, 107. *See also* Exposure techniques in treatment

Flying, fear of. *See* Specific phobia

Forced-thoughts exposures, 144–147. *See also* Exposure techniques in treatment

Friends
changing unhelpful behavior from, 238–241
effect of anxiety on, 234–235
how behaviors by affect the anxiety, 235–238
troubleshooting, 241–242

Friendships, 197–200

Future, fears of, 137. *See also* Worry

Gamma-aminobutyric acid (GABA), 27, 189

Generalized anxiety disorder. *See* Anxiety in general
beliefs often associated with, 30
in children and adolescents (resource list), 252–253
fear of death and, 24
hypochondriasis and, 24
overview, 14, 21–22
relaxation techniques and, 33
resources for, 250–251, 252–253, 253–254

Genetic causes, 26

Geodon (ziprasidone), 187

Germs, fear of, 131

Goal setting, 64–66, 67, 114–117

Graduated exposure, 107. *See also* Exposure techniques in treatment

Half-life of a medication, choosing among medications and, 176–177

Health anxiety, 23–24, 250

Health habits, treatments for anxiety and, 33. *See also* Lifestyle interventions

Health insurance, seeking professional help and, 71

Health issues, 176, 216–219

Heights, fear of. *See* Specific phobia

Herbal treatments, 32, 74, 76, 188–190

Hoarding obsessions/compulsions, 20, 21. *See also* Compulsions; Obsessive-compulsive disorder

Hot flushes, 15, 153

Hyperarousal, posttraumatic stress disorder and, 19

Hypervigilance, 8

Hypochondriasis, 23–24

Ignoring information, 82

Imagery, anxiety-provoking, 86

Images
choosing among treatment strategies, 74–75, 76
examples of, 136–138
exposure techniques and, 33
identifying internal experiences that you fear and avoid, 52, 54–55

Imaginal exposure, acceptance-based treatments and, 169–170

Imagined ugliness, 24

Impulses, anxiety-provoking, 86

Informational causes of anxiety, 29–30

Inheritability of anxiety, 26

Inositol, 190

Instructional causes of anxiety, 29–30

Insurance, seeking professional help and, 71

Internal triggers, 11–12

Internet resources, 246–247

Interoceptive cues. *See* Triggers of anxiety and fear

Interoceptive exercises
acceptance-based treatments and, 169–170
overview, 150–154
when they are not enough, 154–156

Intrinsic reasons for change, 210–211

Kava, 189

Learning as a cause of anxiety, 28–29

Lexapro (escitalopram), 179

Life without anxiety. *See also* Relapse prevention
dealing with relapses, 228, 230, 231
maintaining the progress you've made, 226–228, 229
overview, 221–226, 230, 231–233

Lifestyle interventions
choosing among treatment strategies, 74, 76
diet and nutrition, 195–197
exercise and, 200–202
overview, 33, 195, 206
sleep and, 205–206
social life, 197–200
substance use and, 202–205

Light switches, anxiety concerning, 131

Lightheadedness, panic attacks and, 15

Locks, anxiety concerning, 131

Long-term goals, 65–66

Lorazepam, 185

Lyrica (pregabalin), 186

Manerix (moclobemide), 183–184

Media, causes of anxiety and, 31

Medical conditions, 176, 216–219

Medical professionals, seeking help from, 70–72

Medication treatments
abuse of medications, 204–205
advantages and disadvantages of, 173–174
anti-anxiety medications and, 184–186
anticonvulsants, 186
antidepressants, 178–184
antipsychotics, 187
beta-adrenergic blockers, 186–187
choosing among medications, 175–177
choosing among treatment strategies, 74, 76
decisions regarding, 174
depression and, 209
developing a treatment plan and, 75
effective medication, 177–178
myths and misconceptions regarding, 171–173
overview, 27, 32, 171
psychological problems and, 209
questions and concerns regarding, 188
resources for, 254
seeking professional help and, 70
stages of, 174–175
types of medications, 177–187

Meditation
choosing among treatment strategies, 74, 76
developing a treatment plan and, 75
overview, 33, 190
stress management and, 216

Memories
choosing among treatment strategies, 74–75, 76
examples of, 136–138
exposure techniques and, 33
identifying internal experiences that you fear and avoid, 52, 54–55

Memory, role of, 81–82

Mental illness, as an obstacle to treating your anxiety, 208–209

Messiness, fear of, 131

Mindfulness-based strategies, 169–170, 255. *See also* Acceptance-based treatments

Motivation, 64–65, 209–211

Narcotic use. *See* Drug use

Nardil (phenelzine), 183

Nausea, 14, 153, 154

Needles, fear of
identifying safety behaviors you use with, 52
identifying variables that affect your fear and anxiety and, 40–41
identifying your thoughts associated with, 46
identifying your triggers and, 37

Nervous system responses, fear and, 8–9

Neurontin (gabapentin), 186

Neurotransmitters, 26–27, 179
Nicotine use, 204
Noradrenergic/specific serotonergic
    antidepressants (NaSSA), 181, 182
Norebox (reboxetine), 184
Norepinephrine, 27
Norepinephrine reuptake inhibitors,
    181
Numbness, 15, 152
Nutrition, 195–197

Observational causes of anxiety, 29
Obsessions, 19, 20. See also Obsessive-
    compulsive disorder
Obsessive Compulsive Foundation, 72
Obsessive-compulsive concerns, 36–37,
    40, 45–46
Obsessive-compulsive disorder
    beliefs often associated with, 30
    body dysmorphic disorder and, 24
    fear of death and, 24
    hypochondriasis and, 24
    identifying methods of self-
        protection and, 47, 50, 51–52, 53
    identifying safety behaviors you use
        with, 51
    impulses and, 86
    overview, 13, 19–21
    removing false-safety behaviors and,
        118–123
    resources for, 249–250
Obsessive-compulsive personality
    disorder, 24
Obstacles to treating your anxiety
    choosing among treatment
        strategies, 74, 76
    medical issues and, 216–219
    motivation and, 209–211
    overview, 60, 63–64, 207, 220
    psychological problems and, 208–209
    skill improvement and, 219–220
    stress management and, 212–216
    time issues, 207–208
Omega-3 fatty acids, 190
Open trial of medication, 177
Ordering compulsion, 21. See
    also Compulsions; Obsessive-
    compulsive disorder
Organizations, professional, 71–72
Overinvolvement, emotional, 236–237

Panic attacks, 14–15
Panic disorder
    beliefs often associated with, 30
    fear of death during, 24
    hypochondriasis and, 24
    identifying safety behaviors you use
        with, 51
    identifying variables that affect your
        fear and anxiety and, 40
    identifying your thoughts associated
        with, 45
    identifying your triggers and, 36
    overview, 13, 14–16
    resources for, 248
Paxil (paroxetine), 27, 32. See also
    Medication treatments
Performance anxiety, 9–10, 17. See also
    Social anxiety disorder
Phobia, specific. See Specific phobia
Physical abuse, posttraumatic stress
    disorder and, 18–19
Physical exercise, 200–202
Physical health, 176, 216–219

Physical response
    effects of avoiding, 148–150
    exposure techniques and, 33,
        148–156
    fear and, 9
    identifying, 41, 43, 44
    identifying internal experiences that
        you fear and avoid, 50, 52, 54
Pleasurable activities, stress
    management and, 216
Posttraumatic stress disorder
    beliefs often associated with, 30
    exposure techniques and, 143–144
    imagery and, 86
    memories and, 137
    overview, 13, 18–19
    resources for, 251–252
Pounding heart, 14, 152, 153, 154
Predictions, causes of anxiety and,
    29, 30
Pregnancy, choosing among
    medications and, 176
Preparing for treatment
    challenges and obstacles to, 60,
        63–64
    choosing among treatment
        strategies, 72–75
    developing a treatment plan, 75–76
    finding someone to help and support
        you, 66, 69
    goal setting and, 64–66, 67
    multiple anxiety problems and, 66,
        67–68
    ranking problems to target, 66,
        67–68
    seeking professional help, 70–72
    timing of, 58–64
Probability overestimation, 83
Problem-solving method, 213, 214–215
Professional help, decisions regarding,
    70–72
Professional organizations, 71–72,
    243–246
Progress monitoring, 56, 57. See also
    Self-assessment
Progressive-muscle relaxation,
    158–166. See also Relaxation-based
    treatments
Protection of the self. See Safety
    behaviors
Prozac (fluoxetine), 27, 179
Psychiatrists, seeking help from, 70–72
Psychological causes, 27–31
Psychological problems, as an obstacle
    to treating your anxiety, 208–209
Psychologists, seeking help from, 70–72
Public speaking, exposure techniques
    and, 130

Questioning yourself technique, 96–98

Racing heart
    exposure techniques and, 33
    exposures and, 152, 153, 154
    panic attacks and, 14
Randomized controlled trial (RCT),
    178
Rape, posttraumatic stress disorder
    and, 18–19
Rational thinking technique, 93, 95
Relapse prevention
    choosing among treatment
        strategies, 74, 76
    dealing with relapses, 228, 230, 231

life without anxiety, 221–226
    maintaining the progress you've
        made, 226–228, 229
    medication and, 172, 174
Relationships
    changing unhelpful family behavior
        and, 238–241
    effect of anxiety on, 234–235
    how behaviors by others affect the
        anxiety, 235–238
    as an obstacle to treating your
        anxiety, 208–209
    resources for, 254
    social life and, 197–200
Relaxation-based treatments
    breathing retraining, 166–168
    choosing among treatment
        strategies, 74, 76
    developing a treatment plan and, 75
    overview, 33, 157, 170
    progressive-muscle relaxation,
        158–166
    resources for, 255
    sleep and, 206
    stress management and, 216
Relief, thoughts and, 80
Religious obsessions, 20. See also
    Obsessions; Obsessive-compulsive
    disorder
Repeating compulsion, 21. See
    also Compulsions; Obsessive-
    compulsive disorder
Resources, 243–256
    Internet resources, 246–247
    professional organizations, 243–246
    readings and videos, 248–256
Reuptake process, 26
Rewarding yourself, motivation and,
    211
Risperdal (risperidone), 187
Rules, rigid, 84, 87–88, 100–101

Sadness, thoughts and, 80
Safety behaviors
    alcohol use and, 203–204
    causes of anxiety and, 29, 31
    effect of on family and friends, 235
    external triggers and, 11
    identifying methods of self-
        protection and, 47, 50, 51–52, 53
    panic disorder and, 15
    relapse prevention and, 225
    removing, 118–123
Saving-related obsessions, 20. See also
    Obsessions; Obsessive-compulsive
    disorder
Selective serotonin reuptake inhibitors
    (SSRIs)
    antipsychotics and, 187
    benzodiazepines and, 185–186
    overview, 27, 179–181
Self-assessment
    identifying internal experiences that
        you fear and avoid, 50, 52, 54
    identifying situations and objects
        that you avoid, 47, 49
    identifying variables that affect your
        fear and anxiety, 38, 40–41, 42
    identifying your physical sensations,
        41, 43, 44
    identifying your thoughts, 43, 45–
        47
    importance of, 56
    progress monitoring and, 56, 57

relapse prevention and, 221–226
removing false-safety behaviors and, 120
Self-protection, identifying methods of, 47, 50, 51–52, 53. *See also* Safety behaviors
Separation anxiety disorder, 14, 22
Seroquel (quetiapine), 187
Serotonin, 27, 179
Sexual abuse, assault, or rape, 18–19, 30
Sexual obsessions, 20. *See also* Obsessions; Obsessive-compulsive disorder
Shaking, 14, 154
Shortness of breath, panic attacks and, 14
Short-term goals, 65–66
Shyness
    identifying safety behaviors you use with, 51
    identifying variables that affect your fear and anxiety and, 40
    identifying your thoughts associated with, 45
    identifying your triggers and, 36
Side effects of medications
    benzodiazepines, 185
    choosing among medications and, 176
    myths and misconceptions regarding, 173
    noradrenergic/specific serotonergic antidepressants (NaSSA), 181
    tricyclic antidepressants and, 182
Situational exposure, 32–33
Situational phobias, 18. *See also* Specific phobia
Sleep, 205–206
Smothering sensations, 14, 152, 153, 154
Social anxiety
    exposure techniques and, 128, 130, 132–135
    identifying safety behaviors you use with, 51
    identifying variables that affect your fear and anxiety and, 40
    identifying your thoughts associated with, 45
    identifying your triggers and, 36
    skill improvement and, 219–220
Social anxiety disorder
    beliefs often associated with, 30
    body dysmorphic disorder and, 24
    overview, 13, 16–17
    resources for, 248–249
Social life, 197–200
Social phobia. *See* Social anxiety disorder
Social skills, 219–220
Social support. *See also* Support system
Societal causes, 31
Somatic obsessions, 20. *See also* Obsessions; Obsessive-compulsive disorder
Specific phobia
    beliefs often associated with, 30
    identifying safety behaviors you use with, 52
    identifying variables that affect your fear and anxiety and, 40

identifying your thoughts associated with, 46–47
    identifying your triggers and, 37
    overview, 13, 17–18
    resources for, 251
Stomach pains, 14, 154
Storms, fear of, 131
Stress, as an obstacle to treating your anxiety, 63–64, 212–216
Substance use, 176, 208–209
Substance-induced anxiety disorder, 14, 23
Suicide, medication and, 172
Support system
    changing unhelpful family behavior and, 238–241
    effect of anxiety on, 234–235
    how behaviors by others affect the anxiety, 235–238
    motivation and, 211
    overview, 197–200
    preparing for treatment and, 66, 69–70
Sweating, 14, 153
Symmetry and exactness obsessions, 20. *See also* Obsessions; Obsessive-compulsive disorder

Test anxiety, 24–25
Therapeutic touch, 190
Therapists, seeking help from, 70–72
Thinking patterns, 29
Thought-challenging strategies, exposure techniques and, 114
Thoughts
    causes of anxiety and, 29, 30
    changing, 86–103
    choosing among treatment strategies, 74–75, 76
    examples of, 136–138
    exposure techniques and, 33
    identifying, 43, 45–47, 86–103, 103
    identifying internal experiences that you fear and avoid, 52, 54–55
    overview, 79, 106
    problems you may encounter when working with, 103, 105
    relapse prevention and, 223
    relationship between feelings and, 79–82
    removing false-safety behaviors and, 120, 122, 123
    types of, 82–86, 87, 106
Time involved in treatment, 60, 63, 207–208
Timing of treatment (is now the time?), 58–64
Tingling sensations, 15, 152
Trauma, posttraumatic stress disorder and, 18–19
Trauma-related anxiety
    exposure techniques and, 140–144
    identifying safety behaviors you use with, 52
    identifying variables that affect your fear and anxiety and, 40
    identifying your thoughts associated with, 46
    identifying your triggers and, 37
    resources for, 251–252

Treatment obstacles. *See* Obstacles to treating your anxiety
Treatment plan, 75–76
Treatment preparation. *See* Preparing for treatment
Treatments
    choosing among treatment strategies, 72–75
    developing a treatment plan and, 75–76
    medication, 32
    overview, 31–33
Trembling, 14, 154
Trichotillomania, resources for, 250
Tricyclic antidepressants, 182–183
Triggers of anxiety and fear
    exposure plans and, 110, 111–117
    identifying your triggers, 35–38, 39
    overview, 10–12
    panic attacks and, 15
    relapse prevention and, 222

Ugliness, imagined, 24
Unconscious thoughts, role of, 81
Unsteadiness, panic attacks and, 15
Urges. *See also* Compulsions
    choosing among treatment strategies, 74–75, 76
    examples of, 136–138
    identifying internal experiences that you fear and avoid, 52, 54–55

Valium (diazepam), 32. *See also* Medication treatments
Veterans, posttraumatic stress disorder and, 18–19

War trauma, posttraumatic stress disorder and, 18–19
Washing compulsion, 21. *See also* Compulsions; Obsessive-compulsive disorder
Websites, 246–247
Wellbutrin (bupropion), 184
Withdrawal symptoms from medication, 185
Witnessing violence, posttraumatic stress disorder and, 18–19
Worry
    exposure techniques and, 140–144
    fears of the future, 137
    generalized anxiety disorder and, 21–22
    identifying safety behaviors you use with, 51
    identifying variables that affect your fear and anxiety and, 40
    identifying your thoughts associated with, 45
    identifying your triggers and, 36
    overview, 8
    resources for, 250–251
Worry/trauma script, 140–144. *See also* Exposure techniques in treatment

Yoga, 190

Zyban (bupropion), 184
Zyprexa (olanzapine), 187

About the Authors

Martin M. Antony, PhD, President-Elect of the Canadian Psychological Association, is Professor and Director of Graduate Training in the Department of Psychology at Ryerson University in Toronto. He is also Director of Research at the Anxiety Treatment and Research Centre, St. Joseph's Healthcare, Hamilton, Ontario. An award-winning researcher, Dr. Antony is the coauthor of *When Perfect Isn't Good Enough, 10 Simple Solutions to Panic,* and numerous other books. His research, writing, and clinical practice focus on cognitive-behavioral therapy and the treatment of anxiety disorders. He has been widely quoted in the U.S. and Canadian media.

Peter J. Norton, PhD, is Associate Professor of Psychology at the University of Houston and Director of the University of Houston Anxiety Disorder Clinic. His research on anxiety and its treatment has been honored with awards from the National Institutes of Health and other organizations. The author of over 60 research papers, Dr. Norton has delivered many presentations and workshops for the scientific community, therapists, and the general public.